"Michael Arthur has written a must-read for anyone living with brain injury. I found his book highly relatable and credible. A page turner."

Kevin Sorbo, *a Hollywood actor, is best known as the star of* Hercules. *After sustaining an on-set injury, he found* True Strength *on his own road to recovery.*

Embracing Hope After Traumatic Brain Injury

This important book provides a firsthand account of a university professor who experienced traumatic brain injury. It tells the story of Michael Arthur, who had recently accepted a position as vice principal of a new high school. After only two weeks on the job, he was involved in a car accident while driving through an intersection in northern Utah.

Through his personal account, he takes the reader into the dark interworkings of his mind as he tries to cope with his new reality. He provides insight into how he learned how to process information and even speak without stumbling on his words while also sharing how his significant relationships suffered as he tried to navigate the restless seas of doubt while trying to circumvent his unyielding symptoms.

The book is about finding optimism and gaining insight into the struggles of the brain-injured patient and about trying to understand the perspectives of loved ones who can't quite grasp the idea of an invisible injury. From the sudden onset of garbled speech to the challenges of processing information, the changing dynamic of the author's life is highlighted to help family members and healthcare workers better understand.

Michael S. Arthur completed his doctorate in education at Concordia University in the United States. He currently teaches graduate research courses to teachers working toward their master's degrees in education. After suffering a traumatic brain injury, Michael was determined to learn all he could about post-concussion syndrome to help himself and others.

After Brain Injury: Survivor Stories
Series Editor: Barbara A. Wilson

This new series of books is aimed at those who have suffered a brain injury, and their families and carers. Each book focuses on a different condition, such as face blindness, amnesia and neglect, or diagnosis, such as encephalitis and locked-in syndrome, resulting from brain injury. Readers will learn about life before the brain injury, the early days of diagnosis, the effects of the brain injury, the process of rehabilitation, and life now. Alongside this personal perspective, professional commentary is also provided by a specialist in neuropsychological rehabilitation, making the books relevant for professionals working in rehabilitation such as psychologists, speech and language therapists, occupational therapists, social workers and rehabilitation doctors. They will also appeal to clinical psychology trainees and undergraduate and graduate students in neuropsychology, rehabilitation science, and related courses who value the case study approach.

With this series, we also hope to help expand awareness of brain injury and its consequences. The World Health Organization has recently acknowledged the need to raise the profile of mental health issues (with the WHO Mental Health Action Plan 2013–20) and we believe there needs to be a similar focus on psychological, neurological and behavioural issues caused by brain disorder, and a deeper understanding of the importance of rehabilitation support. Giving a voice to these survivors of brain injury is a step in the right direction.

Published titles:

The Sibling Relationship After Acquired Brain Injury
Family Dynamics Across the Lifespan
Penelope Analytis

For more information about this series, please visit: www.routledge.com/After-Brain-Injury-Survivor-Stories/book-series/ABI

Embracing Hope After Traumatic Brain Injury

Finding Eden

Michael S. Arthur

With contributions from
Dr. Deana Adams

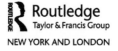
Routledge
Taylor & Francis Group

NEW YORK AND LONDON

Cover Image: Getty Images

First published 2022
by Routledge
605 Third Avenue, New York, NY 10158

and by Routledge
2 Park Square, Milton Park, Abingdon, Oxon, OX14 4RN

Routledge is an imprint of the Taylor & Francis Group, an informa business

© 2022 Michael S. Arthur

The right of Michael S. Arthur to be identified as author of this work has been asserted by him in accordance with sections 77 and 78 of the Copyright, Designs and Patents Act 1988.

All rights reserved. No part of this book may be reprinted or reproduced or utilised in any form or by any electronic, mechanical, or other means, now known or hereafter invented, including photocopying and recording, or in any information storage or retrieval system, without permission in writing from the publishers.

Trademark notice: Product or corporate names may be trademarks or registered trademarks, and are used only for identification and explanation without intent to infringe.

Library of Congress Cataloging-in-Publication Data
A catalog record for this book has been requested

ISBN: 9781032105802 (hbk)
ISBN: 9781032105789 (pbk)
ISBN: 9781003216056 (ebk)

DOI: 10.4324/9781003216056

Typeset in Times New Roman
by Apex CoVantage, LLC

Contents

    of Brain Injury   134

    References   149
    Index   156

Introduction

This important book, *Embracing Hope After Traumatic Brain Injury*, is a firsthand account of a university professor who experienced traumatic brain injury. The author, Michael Arthur, had recently moved his family from Oregon to Utah after accepting a position as vice principal of a new high school. After a great deal of excitement and only two weeks on the job, he was T-boned while driving through an intersection in northern Utah.

Michael was ecstatic about recently earning his doctorate degree and was suddenly thrust into an abyss of uncertainty. Through his personal account in *Finding Eden*, he takes the reader into the dark interworkings of his mind as he tries to cope with his new reality and how to process information and even speak without stumbling on his words. Michael shares his story on how his significant relationships suffered as he tried to navigate the restless seas of doubt while trying to circumvent his unyielding symptoms.

From the sudden onset of garbled speech to the challenges of processing information, the changing dynamic of the author's life is highlighted to help family members and healthcare workers better understand.

Finding Eden is about reconnecting with family and friends and how to embrace hope when life has pressed down hard. It's about finding optimism. It's about gaining insight into the struggles of the brain-injured patient. It's also about trying to understand the perspectives of loved ones who can't quite grasp the idea of an *invisible* injury.

Contributors

Biography (Author)

Michael S. Arthur completed his doctorate in education at Concordia University in the United States. His vocation includes teaching graduate research courses to teachers working toward their master's degrees in education. Michael developed a passion for learning all he could about acquired brain injury after he was broadsided in a traffic accident. His goal is to encourage others who also struggle with post-concussion syndrome.

Biography (Contributor)

Deana Adams, PhD, LPC-S, is the executive director of *Hope Behavioral Health*, a private practice specializing in traumatic brain injury. As the president/founder of *Hope After Brain Injury*, Dr. Adams speaks nationally and internationally, sharing insight into how to effectively counsel and facilitate successful recovery for those affected by brain injury.

Acknowledgments

To Dr. Deana Adams: Thank you from the bottom of my heart for agreeing to partner on this book. With over 25 years of experience as a professional counselor, helping individuals and families who suffer from traumatic brain injury, you have brought incalculable worth to this project. Thank you!

To my very special friend and wife, Kindra: Thank you for your steadfast love and support throughout this challenging season in our lives together. Post-concussion symptoms can be extremely disruptive to a relationship, but your patience and kindness are appreciated more than you could know.

To my incredible daughter, Rachael: Thank you for your willingness to share your real-life story that brought so much pain into your life. You stand as a beacon of hope to so many people around the world who've also lost a loved one in battle and endured the struggles of PTSD.

To my family and friends: Thank you for your incredible support throughout my healing journey over the past few years. Your encouragement throughout the writing of this book not only helped me remember important events but created a work meant to fully support and encourage people who suffer from post-concussion syndrome.

To Dr. Benjamin Nguyen at UT Southwestern Medical Center in Dallas: Your expertise with TBI is exceptional. Your long list of honors is impressive. But mostly, I am thankful for your kindness, genuine empathy, and holistic approach. You make a real difference in the lives of countless patients setting them on a path of hope.

Dr. Deana Adams wishes to thank her beloved husband, Rick, who encourages her passion as the president/founder of Hope After Brain Injury and her devotion to clients in her private practice, Hope Behavioral Health, PLLC.

Deana wishes to thank Dr. Michael Arthur for his perseverance as an mTBI/PCS survivor and his desire to encourage others going through the brain injury journey. She is honored to be invited to write a bit of her expertise. It has been a joy to work with him!

Deana wishes to thank Patti Foster, an amazing TBI survivor who inspired her to start working with the greatest group of men and women on the planet: TBI survivors and their families.

Foreword

Michael Arthur and I became colleagues and friends in 2013 when we each joined the initial doctoral cohort at Concordia University in Portland, Oregon. Being the only Oregonians among the fifteen was part of that; our worldwide online cohort left Mike and me in the same time zone and easily able to communicate in real time. While working very, very hard, we also visited with each other, including in-person, and we continue to be great friends. As Mike learned about me, he discovered that my immediate family has been, and continues to be, profoundly impacted by traumatic brain injury. Additionally, as a teacher, coach, and school administrator, I have worked with dozens of students with native or acquired brain injuries.

Michael and I came to our doctoral studies on different paths. Mine was as a teacher and coach and then as a school administrator, which included special services management. Michael was a blue-collar worker who had been impacted by the recession and found his way to teaching at a community college through a career shift into journalism, broadcasting, and business. Four years later, Mike graduated. As we sat at his graduation dinner with a New Yorker from our cohort, Michael spoke with me about his next steps. I was hearing how his dreams of working with kids were really coming true.

In a few words, it is impossible to describe the intensity of the emotion and intellect I heard at that table. I understood, however, because I had finished earlier and was applying our learned education principles to my work as a superintendent. I shared in the joy of their achievement in a very tangible way; we began together. For several years I had wondered how Michael might find his way into K–12 education; he did not hold a teaching certificate. But I led a total charter district—a single rural K–12 school organized as a charter, so I knew it was theoretically possible. And lo and behold, I was sitting at a table with a charter school director who eventually was going to interview and hire Dr. Arthur for an assistant principal's position in Utah.

In the fall of 2017, Mike was living the dream. He was doing exactly what he believed was possible when he made that radical 2013 decision to leap into education at the doctoral level. For some, though, life has other plans. In this moving personal account, Dr. Michael Arthur describes how his world exploded at an intersection and the full ramifications of the word *accident*. From being sent home from the emergency room until today, Dr. Arthur applies his skills as a qualitative researcher and writer to tell his story. For those who have intimate connections with a person with TBI and for those who do not, this work may help further the understanding of how difficult and how misunderstood living with TBI may be.

Mike began this journey with an ER diagnosis of a concussion before he was sent home after the car crash. The next day, when his speech became garbled, although his thinking was clear, Mr. and Mrs. (Kindra) Arthur realized they would need some immediate follow-up. In the next months, the family rode the TBI roller coaster as doctors disagreed regarding the pathology and Mike manifested more symptoms. Not surprisingly, Dr. Arthur's work was profoundly impacted. As many do, Michael tried to press on, but the injury left him at times unable to write a cogent paragraph or organize a cohesive presentation. He did not understand why he could not interact interpersonally as he did before or move normally.

It took Michael Arthur years to get to a place where he is well, content, and motivated to tell his story so that others do not feel alone. Because Michael *was* alone—he was in a solitary abyss he did not comprehend. At times, depressed, angry, hopeless, and defiant, among other feelings, Michael turned to research and then reached out to find a world of people like him. Online communities and this Routledge series of books were among the tools he used to understand and learn to deal with what was happening and had happened to him. For me, simply, I know my friend is back in a much better head- and heart-space than he was just a few years ago, and I have known those who did not survive those feelings Dr. Arthur is working through and past.

TBI is a lot of things. None would find them pleasant, but TBI does provide an opportunity for change and growth. And at the root, it is the work related to the injury that becomes a part of one's life and being. Although not requested, this work is essential, and its neglect has profound effects. Supported, this work allows an individual to move out of what can be a very dark place into a bright future, with renewed hope and purpose. This is Mike Arthur and his family's story.

Dr. James MacAdam Brookins
School Superintendent, Retired

1

A Moment in Time

Introduction

On the weekend before the accident, our visit to the mountain town of Eden seemed metaphoric on how we were feeling. We had entered a special place, and it was a garden of possibilities. Eden sat in the hill country lying between the north and middle fork of the Ogden River and was home to the Powder Mountain Ski Resort. With the higher elevation and a peaceful lake off in the distance, the small town provided the perfect getaway for falling in love all over again. We strolled a quiet street near an old general store as a gentle breeze rustled the trees and nudged our conversation toward dreams about the future.

We approached a historic building and found a large unlocked door. Most businesses in Utah were closed on Sundays, so we were careful as we entered a smallish-sized room. To our surprise, there was a fully stocked coffee bar with a barista who politely welcomed us in. She had a pleasant smile and didn't say much as we studied the menu behind her. We ordered two lattes and waited as she worked her magic. The drinks were gently crafted and handed to us with the same attention to detail. "That's on the house," she said softly. Noticing us taken aback, she explained that the business was actually closed and she had simply forgotten to lock the door but was happy to serve us.

10.4324/9781003216056-1

The small-town barista represented so many people we'd met in Utah. Most were kind, attentive, and caring. This, too, was adding to our confidence about our new life in this Western US state. I had accepted a position as vice principal of a high school just outside of Ogden. The state of Oregon was our home for many years, but Utah offered more than just a new career. Its awe-inspiring Wasatch Mountains were unfathomable. They exemplified the handiwork of creative genius and spoke their own special language. It wasn't a known dialect but uniquely clear and beautiful.

On the morning of the accident, I had just completed another training for my new position and was making my way across town. As I drove toward that infamous intersection, I noticed a 1940s craftsman-style home that sat on the corner of 30th and Wall. I've always admired the architects of yesteryear and how they toiled working at drafting tables before the dawn of computer-aided design. This particular home sat proud for close to a hundred years but was beginning to show its age. It wasn't the house that encroached the intersection; it was the other way around. The city grew, and so did many of its roads. Unfortunately, the front of the house was positioned very close to the street, obstructing the view for drivers headed eastbound.

As I approached the intersection, the historic home sat immediately to my left, and green lights were just ahead. Nothing seemed out of the ordinary. I've always considered myself a defensive driver and was aware the home created a barrier. It's the risk drivers have to take. This was the case with the home sitting so close to the street; I simply couldn't see the cross traffic and trusted that things would be fine. After all, they've always been fine before. In all my years of driving, I have never witnessed a car blow through a red light and slam into another vehicle. And I had certainly never been involved in that type of collision myself.

I sensed that something was amiss as my car first crossed into the intersection. Through my periphery, I noticed something was out of place. I had just enough time to turn my head ever so slightly, moving my eyes even more. That's when I saw her face. She had a look of confusion but never pressed her brakes. She seemed in another world and not taking into account the brevity of the moment. Although I don't remember every detail of the accident, it still comes to my mind. I've even sat up quickly in the midst of a nightmare, sensing her car rushing toward me. It's always the same scene, her vehicle about to hit mine. That's what I remember most, that brief moment before the accident and bracing for the unknown.

In that very brief moment before the crash, I don't remember being afraid. Everything seemed in living color and hyper-sensitized. I quickly gripped the steering wheel and braced for impact, no matter what that would entail. There wasn't time for fight or flight. There wasn't time to think about my spouse, family, or friends. There certainly wasn't time to call out to God. There was only the immediate circumstance, and I needed to hold on tight. There was an opposing vehicle traveling at full speed, and it was about to hit me. It wouldn't be making contact with the front or rear portions of my car. The vehicle blowing through the intersection was laser-focused at the center of my vehicle and body.

Life has its seasons, and trials can press down hard beyond measure. King Solomon concluded there are times and seasons for everything under heaven. There is a time for weeping and a time for laughing. A time to be silent and a time to speak. There is a time to mourn and a time to dance (The Holy Bible, New International Version [NIV], 1973/2011, Ecclesiastes 3). Everyone experiences the dichotomies of life. No one is exempt from the highs or the lows. The healthy and the not so healthy. Each of us has our own journey, and even car accidents are unique with their own circumstance and outcome. And this was the case in our experience. We had embraced Eden in all of her glory. She was within our reach, and we were ready. It was our determination that a new day had begun in our lives, but we didn't know what lay just ahead.

I remember there was silence for a moment as smoke came through the dash in front of me. The airbags had all deployed, as well, adding to the dramatic scene. After that brief moment of quiet, it was as though a stagehand had moved up the volume, ever so steadily. My heart started to pound harder as I pressed into the door with my shoulder, trying to escape. It was jammed. I quickly crawled over the center console to the passenger door and threw it open. I crawled through the space and stood just outside in disbelief. I had just experienced a serious traffic accident, even being T-boned in my driver's door, and I was alive and standing on the street.

This was not supposed to be part of our Eden experience. When we walked the road in that breathtaking mountain town just two days prior, we were over the moon in our imaginations. We were hopeful and optimistic. Life has challenges, but we did that already. In a seemingly short period of time, we had lost loved ones. We had been sick and suffered financial setbacks. It was assuredly our turn for Eden. I remember whispering my prayer before we even departed for Utah. I asked for a time of respite by the *still waters* spoken of in the Psalms. I made these verses my hope as we left the West Coast and sincerely believed it was our time for something special and new.

After pulling myself from the car, I stood for a minute on the street and took in the scene. There was still smoke coming from my car though it was now faint. It was another surreal movie scene with all characters in place waiting for the director's cue. However, I would not play the protagonist this time but the victim. I was the unsuspecting person instantly removed from his normal way of life for something much different. I wasn't able to see the person who ran the red light, but I could see her vehicle. I also noticed a third vehicle involved in the accident as a man ran toward me to let me know he had called for help. Then, right on cue, as the surreal experience would dictate, I heard the distant sounds of emergency vehicles on their way.

The day was long, but we gathered our emotions and were thankful that I was not hurt badly or even killed. One of the officers at the scene stopped by the hospital to ask some questions. He was surprised to see that I was no worse for wear, given the condition of the other vehicles involved in the crash. We were surprised too. In fact, other than feeling like I had just collided with a football player, I felt OK. I mulled the accident in my mind over and over: I had a green light and was driving through the intersection. There was a historic home blocking my view. A vehicle ran through a red light and slammed into mine. It was a direct hit. I was T-boned at full speed and had no real injuries to show for it. These were my thoughts for days to come.

Tragic events have a way of instilling retrospection in the soul. On the day following my accident, I waxed philosophical as we drove past the state capitol building. Somehow, the grandeur of the structure and my recent near-death experience prompted me toward a conversation about life and its brevity and ultimate significance. This was the backdrop during my first encounter with what could be referred to as a brain-mouth disconnect. When

I tried to speak, my words became garbled and unintelligible. I remember pointing toward the architecture as I tried to make my point, but it was the precise moment I fumbled every word. It was a nerve-racking experience that prompted us to call our doctor right away.

When I was a teenager, I had the opportunity to visit my good friend who lived in a big city, about five hours from my home. David Johnston had a great sense of humor and was always at the top of his class. I spent a week with him at his folks' house over one summer break. On a Saturday night, we decided to take a stroll to the nearest convenience store. We thought ourselves highly advanced linguists and loved to make up silly words, like "sweave," a combination of "swerve" and "weave." While maybe not the usual sort of fun for teens barely 16 years old, it was important to us. We spent countless hours twisting the English language to fit our ideas on how the world should communicate. Being able to articulate well was important to David and me. Not that we would ever attain the eloquence of William Shakespeare, but it was our lofty goal. When I think back to that night, David and I laughed so hard, we cried; it was all related to word usage. And now that my words were escaping me, it was a very big deal. Word retrieval, or word finding, is one of the common challenges for people who've suffered specific types of brain injury. Especially if one is injured while driving a vehicle, it's the left hemisphere or the frontal and temporal lobes that are commonly affected. I would later learn that when patients like me have trouble speaking, it's because that specific part of the head has been hurt.

The loss of intelligible words was the first sign that I might have been hurt worse than originally thought. My word finding wasn't merely a brief experience that came and went like the kurinji shrub of south India. The stumbling became increasingly common over the coming weeks and months. It was a disconcerting experience that permeated our concerns and gave rise to a growing list of questions, such as the following: If I did have a "mild" TBI, or concussion, how long would it last? If most football players recover quickly from concussions, would I do the same? Why do I stumble on my words and most football players don't? Can a person die from a "mild" TBI? What happens if someone sustains a second concussion not long after the first? Are medications available that help with the speech? How soon would I be able to return to full-time work?

Still not knowing much about my injury, the symptoms became increasingly noticeable as time moved on. I was having unbearable headaches, which one healthcare worker referred to as nothing more than a migraine that *may* or *may not* be attributed to the accident. I left the appointment even more confused than before. I knew intuitively that the pain I was experiencing, which began just hours after the accident, was a direct result of the crash. I wondered why someone would make such a statement. Even if it were true, it wouldn't be helpful to a patient experiencing multiple symptoms immediately following a traumatic event. Unfortunately, most of my questions remained unanswered for several months after the accident. Through my own research and experience, I now know that my response was common among individuals who've experienced a traumatic event. It simply takes time, research, and advice from a good medical team to become more familiar with head injuries and how to respond.

TBIs, even those classified as "mild," have the potential to bring about a great many concerns for the patient. And depending on the mechanism of injury even a mild TBI, can be time-consuming and difficult to treat. Researchers at Monash University Accident Research Center in Melbourne found that side-impact car crashes, such as the one I experienced, tend to have more devastating effects on the human body than any other type of vehicle crash (2020). That's not to overstate this type of accident above a head-on collision or rollover, only that when a vehicle is broadsided at full speed or even slower than full speed, the consequences can be devastating to the occupants within the broadsided vehicle.

I was eventually diagnosed as having a mild TBI. Unfortunately, the word use of "mild" often causes confusion among employers, fellow workers, schoolteachers, administrators, and others who might have a vested interest in your well-being. The symptoms and long-term consequences of a "mild" TBI can be anything but mild or inconsequential. In my case, in addition to severe headaches, I was experiencing pressure near my temporal areas and across my forehead. I was also experiencing difficulty concentrating and had some short-term memory issues.

In the early months following my accident, I learned the importance of assembling a team of medical professionals who specialize in TBIs. This point became especially clear after I experienced a horrible reaction to a specific medication. As directed, I took the prescription just before going to bed, and everything seemed fine as I slipped into a sound sleep. Then, just after midnight, I began to wake and slowly opened my eyes. Something wasn't right. I turned my head and looked about the room as the nightlight illumined buckling lines and moving walls. The room was still mostly dark, but I could make out its walls and how they were now dancing out of rhythm. No longer did the floor, walls, or ceiling retain their submissive roles. They were now encroaching upon each other and moving desperately about the room. I was scared out of my mind and quickly made my way to the living area.

My heart was racing as the living room walls began to close in on me. I quickly paced the floor, back and forth. My skin felt clammy and warm. The walls continued their march toward me, closer and closer. I literally wanted to die at that moment because my perception of reality was out of control. It's as though I couldn't control my thoughts. They were rampant and doing their own thing, not making sense in my head. Every time I tried to create or control a thought, it escaped into a vapor. My heart pounded ever faster and faster. And when I felt the cliff getting ever so close, I ran back to my wife, who drove me to a nearby hospital emergency room.

My response to the medication is difficult to describe and more frightening than anything I had ever experienced. I don't place blame on the doctor who prescribed the medication, but I was determined, more than ever, to assemble a medical team specifically trained in head trauma. Post-concussion syndrome (PCS) can be highly disruptive to a person's life, and it certainly has been in mine. When we walked the awe-inspiring town of Eden just before the accident, we were hopeful. Eden, with her rolling hills and gentle spirit, became our symbol of a better day. She was where we would reside in our hearts and became our metaphor of hope. It was our turn to let the embers of life cool as we sat by the quiet waters of restoration. This was our conversation as we strolled Eden's picturesque landscape, but an accident just two days later set us on a new and unexpected course.

A hopeful heart can become your reality even if you've suffered a TBI and the PCS that can follow. The days might be dark and gloomy, but it's the sunrise that keeps us going. The darkness won't overcome those who embrace that life has its seasons, and winter doesn't stay around forever. Beyond the post-concussion symptoms, there is still the warmth of a rising sun with its majesty and message of another day. In time, its rays will penetrate our imaginations and teach us the meaning of hopefulness. It is in that place that one finds stillness and peace. For it's in that quiet place where the soul can truly be restored.

Eden has mostly remained a garden of hope for me in spite of my accident on that autumn afternoon in northern Utah. But there are days when the symptoms press in harder and harder, and hope seems to fade into an abyss of fear and doubt. When I've struggled, Eden, in all her glory, escapes me and is nowhere to be found. J. M. Coetzee's translation of Ina Rousseau's poem, "Somewhere in Eden," describes a very special garden also distant from her original purpose:

> Somewhere in Eden, after all this time,
> does there still stand, abandoned, like
> a ruined city, gates sealed with grisly nails,
> the luckless garden?
>
> Is sultry day still followed there
> by sultry dusk, sultry night,
> where on the branches sallow and purple
> the fruit hangs rotting?
>
> Is there still, underground,
> spreading like lace among the rocks
> a network of unexploited lodes,
> onyx and gold?

Through the lush greenery
their wash echoing afar
do there still flow the four glassy streams
of which no mortal drinks?

Somewhere in Eden, after all this time,
does there still stand, like a city in ruins,
forsaken, doomed to slow decay,
the failed garden?

As our light of hope seemed to fade behind the Wasatch Mountains, we finally determined that the beautiful state of Utah might not be our final destination. We needed another "new beginning," a place where our little family could not only start over but flourish. As my wife had done in previous years, she encouraged a move to her former home in the southern United States. As a young resident of Texas, she experienced the wide-open spaces and hospitality the state was famous for. She was doing more than just hinting about a move this time; she was adamant that we seriously consider the possibility. We definitely needed another fresh start, so we rented a truck, packed our belongings, and headed out on our new adventure.

2

New Beginning

The sun had barely risen over our Utah home when our friend Gary Turman started the ignition on our rented truck to let it warm. He was our long-time friend and flew up from Texas to lead our small caravan to our new home in Georgetown, about 1,300 miles to the south. I was a passenger in the trailing vehicle and sat quietly as we drove adjacent to the Wasatch Mountains. These were the same majestic mountains cradling the tiny town of Eden that called out to us on that weekend before the accident. Even though we had faced so many challenges, the mountains still proclaimed their message of hope. Their peaks reached upward and called us to do the same. The psalmist states, "Day after day they pour forth speech; night after night they reveal knowledge" (Psalm 19:2, NIV), and we understood our decree. It was one of hope in finding our own Eden beyond the mountains of Utah.

My wife, Kindra, often shared stories about the wide-open range and big blue skies of Texas. She lived there before we were married and desperately wanted to return one day. There was plenty to do in the large cities, but the old country was never far away with farmlands, horses, trail rides, fishing, and lots and lots of land. She talked about the ranches and places to visit, like the Alamo and the state capitol. The Fort Worth Stockyards was especially notable and represented the best of Texas. There were long-horned steers, dancing, outdoor festivities, and plenty of barbecues. Texans took great pride in their state and would never play second fiddle to another.

Gary was determined and pressed on toward Texas no matter the weather or other eventuality. We drove mile after mile through sunshine, pouring rain, sleet, and even snow. At one point, we drove over a peak above 9,000 feet with blistering winds pushing hard against the truck. For me, someone with PCS, the trip was daunting and we needed Gary's raw grit. After all, as a former police officer for a very large department, he had learned the meaning of perseverance. Truth be told, Gary had impressive tenacity since the time we first met back when we were in junior high school. It was part of his character, his DNA. It was his toughness that would get us to our new destination safely, on time, and without incident.

When you have a friend like Gary, there are many double-takes through the years. I remember the first time I was taken aback by Gary. We were still in high school and took some buddies with us to the historic town, Tule Lake, in the Pacific Northwest of the United States. The town was known for its national monument, the Tule Lake War Relocation Center. It was one of ten concentration camps built in 1942 to incarcerate Japanese Americans after they were forcibly removed from their homes. It was an incredibly sad blot in American history, and we wanted to pay our respects. There were also famous caves in the area, including the Catacomb system that drew our attention. We came well prepared with maps, flashlights, jackets, and food. We figured extra food would be a good plan in case of a wrong turn in the winding cave system.

Tule Lake was a several hours' drive from our home, so we rented a room for the night. We stayed smack-dab in the middle of town in a room above a local eatery. I remember a long creaky hallway with a few doors to the left and right. Our room overlooked the dead-quiet street below. We had such a great time laughing and staying up through the little wee hours of the morning, sharing jokes that didn't make sense or were a little off-color. Gary and another friend lit up some old stogies right there in the hotel room. Our trip was both educational and fun. But the thing that stands out most in my mind and sets Gary apart from the others in our group took place on our way home from Tule Lake. With one act of decisiveness and compassion, Gary solidified his place as the unofficial leader of our group.

We were headed back in two vehicles through the high desert region of eastern Oregon when a deer jumped out in front of the lead car. It happened so quickly, there was no way to avoid the collision. As I think back, the unexpected nature of it all seems eerily similar to my T-bone accident. There are times in life when an escape route is simply not possible. That's what happened on our way home from Tule Lake. We were on a long stretch of desert highway and were the only vehicles on the road. Then suddenly, a deer jumped out from a patch of shrubbery and into our path. We slammed on the brakes, but there simply wasn't enough time to stop. It was a very sad experience as the deer was thrown to an area adjacent to the eastbound lane of the roadway.

The other friend and I quickly rushed over to the deer. We felt horrible and didn't know what to do, as we stood motionless and confused. The deer was struggling for air, and there simply was no credible way to save its life. Then, suddenly, we heard the slamming of a car door behind us. We looked back and watched as Gary made his way toward the deer and carrying a gun. "Move back, boys!" he exclaimed with all authority. We quickly moved aside and watched as he put the deer out of its suffering. One clean shot and the deer was at peace. Gary didn't enjoy the experience whatsoever. It wasn't his bid for attention or an opportunity to display his fascination for the Wild West. It was just something that needed to happen quickly, and Gary was one to do it.

Gary has always been a realist, and his decisiveness is a true testament to his character. He had sized up the situation in a matter of a few seconds. We were traveling through the desert. There was no one else on the highway. Civilization was miles away. The deer was suffering and would not survive. For Gary, there was only one solution, and it needed to happen straight away. This was the exact type of decisive leadership Kindra and I needed during our long haul from Utah to Texas. We were overwhelmed, and I was especially symptomatic from the head injury. We needed Gary's no-nonsense approach to lead us through the mountains, across the plains, and to our new home in central Texas. For us, that would be our promised land, and Gary would lead us out of the desert.

Traveling is not easy for someone with PCS. Maybe it has something to do with the constantly changing environment, the movement mile after mile. The brain is an incredibly complex soft organ that functions as the coordinating center of sensation and intellectual and nervous activity. When it's injured to some degree, even if the extent is determined as "mild," movement from one place to another can cause symptoms to be more severe. This was my situation as we journeyed farther and farther south. We were chalking up the miles, and my brain was chalking up the symptoms. I was disoriented and had a hard time processing information. My words were coming out garbled, and I couldn't track with the most basic conversation.

We finally made it to the northern border of Texas with less than 600 miles to go. Gary continued leading the charge in our oversized moving truck and tackling the miles, one by one. Somewhere around midafternoon on the second day, we pulled into a mini-mart gas station. By now, my symptoms were spinning out of control, making the trip much more challenging for me. In addition to pain at both temporal areas, my forehead felt numb, and there was discomfort at two areas at the back of my head. After Kindra parked the car, I tried to hide how I was feeling as she made her way to Gary, who was just now exiting the driver's cab of the truck. I headed into the store.

It was a typical mini-mart one would find along a lonely stretch of highway. There were only two gas lanes and not much available inside the store. For me, it didn't matter because I was on an important mission. As I made my way past the clerk, I looked over and asked where I might find the bathroom. He pointed in one direction, but for some inexplicable reason, I headed in the other. I don't understand why I turned in the opposite direction, but somehow, in the midst of my unbearable symptoms, my brain processed his directions incorrectly. No doubt, the clerk noticed I was mentally off. Maybe he thought I was drunk, on drugs, or overmedicated from a prescription. Who knows? But it didn't help when he raised his voice for others in the store to hear "Hey, Einstein, I pointed in the other direction!" I was too exhausted to be embarrassed. I simply turned, headed down the aisle, and took care of business.

Head-injured patients with persistent PCS often experience a host of symptoms, including headache, extreme noise and light sensitivity, dizziness, irritability, fatigue, anxiety, depression, sleep difficulties, and problems with memory, concentration, and appetite. Of course, there are many similarities from one person to the next, but symptoms can present with their own frequency and level of intensity. In my situation, my greatest struggles have been mostly related to head pain, pressure, fatigue, anxiety, and memory issues. Add to this scenario a long-distance move, and my symptoms will intensify, lasting days or even weeks.

Our move from one state to another triggered my symptoms to level nine on a ten scale. Be it the stress of the move, loading of the truck, or traveling the hundreds of miles. Maybe it was all of the above? Each of the symptoms was present and overtaking my entire being. My headache, along with the other symptoms, hovered at level nine, bringing about depression and a sense of hopelessness. It's during those times that a place called Eden seems elusive and hard to imagine. Eden represented hope for us and was supposed to be a place of rest when life pressed down hard. But when the symptoms become so severe that they envelop every cell in your body, the entirety of who you are, Eden seems nothing more than an obscurity in a faraway land.

> Eden, oh beautiful Eden. Where are you when the trials of life press in? Where are you when there's nothing left to say? Nothing left to do? Are you real or just a fantasy? Will you offer hope again? Where are your pomegranates with their beautiful clusters? What about your grapes with their long stringy vines? Where did you go, my Eden? Beautiful, beautiful, Eden. I called

out, but you didn't answer. I looked everywhere but I'm left feeling hopeless and confused.

People who struggle with PCS need a peaceful environment, a place where they can heal. Moving to Georgetown was a good place for us to start all over again. Stress seemed to most always bring about my headaches, confusion, and irritability. Georgetown represented many new possibilities and changed our outlook for the future. We rented a place on the south side of town that was peaceful and serene and had a down-home feel about it. There was a walking path that worked its way through landscaped grass, well-placed rocks, and newly planted trees. A gentle breeze often blew through the area, making daily walks a real pleasure. It was perfect for peaceful living in a well-designed community complete with ponds, benches, and bluebonnet wildflowers. The bluebonnets, prairie verbena, and blackfoot daisies seemed to be everywhere we looked. The place became our welcome sanctuary following some very tying months.

On one Saturday evening, Kindra and I decided to take our Alaskan Klee Kai for a walk. Akaira loved going out, and we were headed toward her favorite path. The hot Texas sun had already settled for the evening as we neared the final turn on the path. Straight away, Akaira spotted a small rabbit standing close to a nearby fence that ran adjacent to the street. Puppies are easily distracted, and our dog was no different. Weighing in at less than ten pounds and looking exactly like a miniature husky, she pulled for all she was worth. After all, that's what huskies do; they love to pull things. Akaira believed she was as big as any other dog, and the local rabbits reinforced that misconception. She pulled as though she were trying out for the annual Iditarod Sled Dog Race in Anchorage, Alaska!

Kindra and I laughed as she gripped the leash tighter, with Akaira now on her two back legs, pulling even harder. That's the very moment when we heard what sounded like a sprinkler system kicking in behind us. Like two actors in a well-rehearsed musical, we turned in unison, then looked to the ground. There before us, not three feet away, was the largest rattlesnake we'd ever seen. It was long, thick, coiled, and ready to strike! In reality, we could have reached down to touch the snake without taking a single step. I remember glancing at a hiking magazine a few years ago with directions on what to do if one comes across a rattlesnake unexpectedly. I don't recall that running was an option while being so close, but that's exactly what we did. From the very depths of my being, I shouted firmly and loudly, "Run!"

I never imagined that we could run as fast as we did. We ran and ran until we could run no more. Akaira was clearly amused and having a good time, but this was not about her. It was about two grown adults behaving like little school-children. In one fell swoop, the rattlesnake transformed us into Olympian 100-meter-dash runners, a career lasting just a few seconds. And after we were nearly out of breath, we stopped to collect ourselves and reassess the situation. It was a made-for-television moment that rarely comes in life. Our labored breathing eventually turned to laugher. We laughed so hard our eyes filled with tears and even ran down our cheeks. That's when Kindra stated, "Do you think we outran that thing?" After a brief pause, we picked up the dog and ran all the way home.

Laughter is good medicine, especially when life brings its challenges. The rattlesnake experience should have been a tipping point after so many trials and tribulations, but it became a soothing medicine for our souls. We had unexpectedly placed ourselves in a dangerous situation, but it became a teachable moment, another opportunity for introspection. Through the experience, we once again learned the value of genuine laughter from deep within ourselves. We began to understand the significance of allowing ourselves some humor, even when unexpected hardships come our way.

Suffering from the debilitating effects of PCS weighs heavy on the soul. The healing process might be slow for some and slower for others, but even one day of relief from the symptoms can bring enough rejuvenation to make it through another day or even two. If there are more than a few days of relief, that's even better, providing more opportunities to heal. Our new surroundings gave us a sense of normalcy that we craved. Throw in a humorous bout with a rattlesnake, and we were beginning to see a faint light at the end of a very long tunnel. Like many people who've suffered from a head injury, it took me some time to accept that my life would be different from it was before the accident. That's not to say that I will not make good strides in my recovery but that I'll need to adjust to the way things are now in this season of my life. My PCS has persisted for a few years, but I've learned how to mitigate the symptoms by adapting and slowing down to appreciate my family and friends. It's part of a holistic approach that includes an excellent team of medical professionals, exercise, time spent in the great outdoors, and of course, quality time with family and friends.

One of my closest friends used to be one of my professors. Dr. Lori Sanchez was the director of the master's in education program at the university I attended. There was something very special about Lori that my wife and I spotted very early on. Not only did she have an impressive work ethic, she was one of the smartest people we'd ever met. But even more remarkable than her work ethic and acumen was her genuine kindness. We were drawn to her and eventually became the best of friends, sharing our most important life events. From marriages to loss of loved ones to even TBIs, our friendship has never waned. A plaque on my mother's kitchen wall sums our friendship with Lori quite well: "A friend is the one who comes in when the whole world has gone out."

We were all settled into our new Georgetown home when Lori rang us up on the cell phone. She wanted to share some good news that she and her husband, Mike, would be flying to our area as part of annual training for his job. Mike worked in a highly technical field that required adeptness at his craft and a commitment to ongoing training. Lori was excited to share that she'd be coming along and wondered if we could all spend some time together. And spend time together, we did. We toured the foremost sites, ate at fancy restaurants, and visited a funky donut shop complete with a "create your own toppings" option from a particularly weird menu. We had so much fun I nearly forgot about my PCS and forged ahead in spite of the pain. The visit even included a serious conversation about my struggles since the accident and our plans for the future.

Psychologists have concluded that the need to belong is a fundamental element of well-adjusted and happy people. Having friends like Mike and Lori, who know how to bring out your very best self, is crucial in the healing process for anyone with a head injury. One study out of Harvard Medical School included 5,000 participants over a 20-year period. The researchers found one person's happiness can affect an entire social group, "even up to three degrees of separation," and lasts up to one year. Also, we can turn to our friends when we're feeling weary and simply need a dose of optimism. Having friends in one's life improves overall health and even helps people live longer, according to researchers.

Jennifer Abbasi, a managing news editor for the *Journal of the American Medical Association*, stated that having a social support group is crucial for a variety of reasons. The person who stays connected or *socially integrated* is more likely to keep up an exercise plan for the long term and even experience fewer struggles with memory decline. Further, people who make it their ambition to be with others often *ward off* depression and suicide in their quest to stay connected. The contrast, according to Abbasi, is that lonely people have "higher blood pressure and other risk factors for heart disease, and they're more likely to 'give up' or 'quit trying' or deal with a stressor [such as the effects of PCS]."

Good friends provide an emotional salve to the person with a head injury. PCS often brings about depression and anxiety as part of a palette of struggles. These particular symptoms can be extra troublesome because they make you want to disengage and stay secluded far more than is healthy. Meeting up with friends is also important because it reconnects the brain-injured patient with his or her inner self. Close friends know the real you. They notice when you are trying to "hide" or are feeling uncomfortable. Trustworthy friends, who genuinely care about you, know just the right words to encourage and help you to cope. The timely and wise words of a friend bring welcome relief when the symptoms are most challenging. I will always cherish our visit with Mike and Lori as one of our more special times together. In spite of my PCS, which included levels seven and eight head pain, difficulty concentrating, and stumbling of words, every moment was precious.

Most everyone has *friends*, but it's usually a small group that makes up what can be referred to as an *inner circle*. These are the individuals whom you trust implicitly with your deepest thoughts, concerns, hopes, and dreams. Without the love, care, and concern of close family and friends, those who become your closest confidants, there is an increased possibility of anxiety, depression, and hopelessness. And for the person suffering from PCS, the hopelessness can run even deeper. This is precisely how I felt for several months after my traffic accident. I felt alone and hopeless. In fact, until Mike and Lori showed up, I spent untold hours wallowing in the darkness, not knowing how to overcome.

Though hard to explain, perhaps the darkness that surrounds the cave explorer might come close. In the United States, there is a cave system in southern Oregon located about 20 miles from the small town of Cave Junction. Formed in marble, cave passages total more than 15,000 feet, part of the Klamath and Siskiyou mountains. One of the memories a visitor takes away from the inner cave experience is the deep, deep darkness. For just a moment, the tour guide asks that all forms of light be extinguished. There is not even the smallest break, spark, or flicker of light anywhere. The cave darkness is so smothering it envelops your skin and reaches deep into your very soul. Then, after a few seconds, the tour guide allows the light to return, little by little. Even the smallest tinge of light threatens the very existence of the darkness. The blackness scurries away like a frightened capybara.

No one should dwell in the darkness indefinitely. Find a way out. Push against the symptoms and break into the light. The darkness will win without a willingness to overcome it. Do not give up! Resist and fight like never before. There is hope, and you can overcome your struggles with time and practice. Stand up, reach out, and follow the light. Learn what has worked for others who've suffered like you. What did they do to escape the darkness? How did their journey end? Compare those people with others who did not reach out for help. How did their journey end? Make your ambition to overcome. It's not easy, but what alternative is there? Outside of hope, there is no peace. There is no comfort. There is no joy. Reach out to your confidants, those whom you love and trust. If it has been a while, reach out anyway. Meet for coffee. Go for a walk. Whatever it takes to get out of your own head.

Even if you have an excellent support group, the days of discouragement will still come. The symptoms are just too powerful to stay optimistic indefinitely. That is why it's recommended that a counselor, one who advises patients with similar struggles, be brought into the conversation. Certainly, close friends bring immeasurable worth to your life, but a counselor knowledgeable about TBI will be value added by providing a more holistic approach to your healing. In addition to the extensive training they've received, they understand the implications and nuances of head injuries that family and friends may not. Professional faith-based counselors can also be excellent counselors, but it's important to find someone with expertise related to your specific struggles.

When I experienced the deep darkness that accompanies PCS, I reached out to a counselor. I found her to be very knowledgeable on head injuries and PCS in particular. She had a kind and respectful demeanor, which helped me feel comfortable sharing my inner struggles from the first day. It's normal to feel as though you can handle things on your own even though you've gone through such an indescribable life experience. In my case, I gave myself a myriad of reasons for not contacting a counselor.

But I soon realized that my doctor was right. A counselor would be hugely helpful as a part of a holistic approach, one that includes every possible tool for success.

After TBI, new beginnings don't come without their own challenges. Gary led us to our new homeland, over a thousand miles from my accident. It was our opportunity to start fresh, and we were ready. My car accident had a dramatic effect on virtually every aspect of my life, including health, relationships, and even employment. But with an excellent healthcare team, supportive family and friends, and a counselor who was knowledgeable about head injuries and PCS, I have made strides toward my end goal for healing and a better life. Though the path has not been easy, not by a long shot, I have made progress in my own healing journey, and you can too. Whatever comes your way, be willing to fight the good fight. Know that there are others ahead of you who have blazed the trail and have done very well. Seasons come and go. And oh, what beauty awaits those who look for spring! Here is a hopeful poem by Evaleen Stein (1863–1923) that tells of spring and how it's just around the corner:

Budding Time Too Brief

O little buds, break not so fast!
The Spring's but new.
The skies will yet be brighter blue,
And sunny too.
I would you might thus sweetly last
Till this glad season's overpast,
Nor hasten through.

It is so exquisite to feel
The light warm sun;

To merely know the Winter done,
And life begun;
And to my heart no blooms appeal
For tenderness so deep and real,
As any one

Of these first April buds, that hold
The hint of Spring's
Rare perfectness that May-time brings.
So take not wings!
Oh, linger, linger, nor unfold
Too swiftly through the mellow mould,
Sweet growing things!

And errant birds, and honey-bees,
Seek not to wile;
And, sun, let not your warmest smile
Quite yet beguile
The young peach-boughs and apple-trees
To trust their beauty to the breeze;
Wait yet awhile!

Evaleen Stein,
Poems in the Waiting Room
(spring, 2020)

3

Coping With Change

After settling in our new home and feeling more optimistic about the future, I interviewed before a hiring board at a nearby community college. In preparing for the big day, I was given a choice of topics for a mini-lesson I'd teach before the group of college administrators. It was a demonstration of sorts to provide a better picture of my teaching ability. I was hopeful because my symptoms had settled, giving me a much better shot at the job. The presentation could not have gone better. I incorporated the latest presentation technology into the lesson and didn't stumble a single word. Even the question-and-answer period after the lesson went exceptionally well. I could feel the excitement bubbling inside me, but I needed to keep my composure. After completing the lesson, the managers excused me from the room, and I headed around a mezzanine to a nearby elevator. That's when I heard someone shouting my name. One of the hiring managers had rushed out of the interview room and met me by the elevator. I was offered the position on the spot and given instructions on what to do next.

I made my way out of the building and couldn't hold back a smile. It was a surreal experience that lifted my spirits higher than they'd been in a very long time. After everything we'd been through following the accident,

10.4324/9781003216056-3

somehow another door had opened with an opportunity for a fresh start and a new classroom. In just a few short weeks, I'd be standing in front of a group of adult learners and teaching the fundamentals of attending college. It wasn't an advanced course, but it provided an excellent opportunity to ease slowly back into the profession. Teaching the entry-level course would be a great place to start as the healing process continued. It would provide a gauge of sorts, or a baseline, to keep an eye on my improvement.

I couldn't wait to get back to the classroom after a head injury and long hiatus. As a family, we were feeling much better about all the positive developments and believed we were finally on a good path. After dealing with the symptoms, month after month, there seemed to be a flicker of light off in the distance. In some ways, teaching paralleled my previous career as a news director in radio broadcasting. I was once again connecting with people and providing important information. Both careers also nurtured growth in my own life. Each provided an opportunity to step out of my comfort zone and into something that could potentially have a positive impact on the lives of others.

Before being hired to work with his spouse on a national radio program with millions of listeners, my brother was employed as an announcer, or DJ, for a popular radio station in our hometown. Dan had a great sense of humor, with a unique twist of sarcasm, which made him a favorite among listeners. I was working at the local plywood mill plugging out thousands of knotholes in sheets of veneer, five days a week. Our parents taught us the importance of a good work ethic, so I appreciated having steady employment. It was a good job that paid the bills, but I was restless and wanted something more. Our family had a long history of working in the plywood mills, so when Dan proved success was possible away from the band saws, lift trucks, and layup lines, I decided to follow his lead. So after a great deal of planning, Kindra and I became full-time college students in search of our own fulfilling careers.

College was a wonderful experience and provided the tools we needed, but I couldn't stop thinking about the radio business. Broadcasting had been my passion since high school, and I even registered to be one of the disc jockeys at the school. It was in our blood, and Dan was already experiencing some success in the field. So when he offered to help me make a *demo tape* for a news anchor position, I said, "Absolutely!" Within a few weeks, I was able to land a position as news director for a small market radio station not far from home. The position seemed to be a perfect fit. They liked the demo and were willing to train me to bring me up to speed. This would be my first opportunity to work in a bona fide radio station, and I couldn't wait.

My new boss, also known as a program director, had been working in the field for several years. He had learned his craft well and was an expert in all areas of broadcasting. I remember hearing him on the radio back when I was in high school. He was well known and already a favorite among the townsfolk. Like any excellent on-air personality, he had more energy than most people and the kind of voice that melded perfectly over the FM radio waves. Even in high school, I recognized that becoming a good radio broadcaster would require more than an outgoing personality. It would require someone who is engaging, well-read, and community-focused and fully understands the complexities of operating a radio broadcasting station.

When I first became interested in broadcasting, there was no World Wide Web providing an open door for just about anyone interested in starting their own broadcasting station, podcast, or another venue. Radio, television, and newspapers were the big three creating a massive, competitive environment for countless individuals who wanted to become a broadcaster or journalist. The good that came from such a restrictive environment was incredibly talented personalities who enjoyed a higher level of notoriety, bigger paychecks, and larger audiences. The downside was that most young people wanting to enter the field simply couldn't.

When I finally got my break in the radio business, my program director had already been in the industry for several years. He was a hard worker and expected the same from his employees. His goal for me was that each word be pronounced correctly and with the proper intonation. There was no room for mistakes as each second in radio was precious. Also, the competitive nature of broadcasting set the bar extremely high for professionalism and likability. Not only was there an intellectual component, there was also the need for an outgoing personality with which the audience could connect. The expectations, even for small- and medium-sized markets, seemed almost insurmountable, but I was determined to make it work. After all, I had made it work while taking a radio course in high school, so I would not have a problem on a live station, or so I thought.

On my first day at the job, I stood behind the microphone in what people in the radio business refer to as a control room. It reminded me of a cockpit in a large aircraft with controls, knobs, and interactive screens everywhere. And there I was, a novice to keep the "aircraft" aloft. My job description included delivering the news at the beginning and midway point, or top and bottom, of each hour. In the interim, I made sure programming, commercials, and public service announcements played on cue during each "block" of the morning. If that weren't enough, I also hosted a 30-minute talk show that followed my final newscast each morning. For a new employee in training, it was a lot to digest.

My program director was seated off to my right near a guest microphone. His purpose wasn't to join me on the airwaves but to coach me through the process. I was excited but also extremely nervous. His was a trial-by-fire teaching approach that expected incremental but steady progress. The second hand on the clock was ticking down to *live air*, which meant it was *go time*. Each morning, I was required to arrive early, sometimes before 4:00 a.m., to research and write the news stories. And now, it was time to deliver what I had written but with accuracy and a level of flair. "Three, two, one . . . you're on the air!" I took a deep breath, looked at the now lit "On Air" sign, and began to read the news.

I did everything wrong. I read the script too fast. I read it too slow. I mispronounced words. My inflection was off. Nothing was going right, but I made it through the first segment and went to a commercial break. "Mike, look at me," my program director exclaimed. "Just calm down and think about what you're doing. You've got twenty seconds left. Put your hand on the microphone switch so you'll be ready." He was very direct but kind. He wanted to see improvement on the very next read. Then because time waits for no one, not even an employee in training, the commercial break ended. This time, however, I was so nervous, I hit all the wrong buttons. It was a clear indication to me that I needed to give up—and give up now.

I tossed my headset on the table and did something I'd never done before; I quit a job while still in training. After all, it was obvious that I didn't have what it took to be a professional broadcaster. I didn't have the skill or talent needed to represent the radio station in providing local and regional news. My long-time dream of entering the radio industry had come to a screeching halt, and it was entirely my fault. My program director had taken time to listen to my demo tape, interview me, and now train me. I had become a disappointment and was indescribably embarrassed. Not realizing the microphone was still on, I looked at my boss and said, "I can't do this," and made my way to the back of the room to take a seat. Unfortunately, when I sat on the barstool, it actually broke. It broke loudly, and it broke thoroughly. It was a rare trifecta of failure. I failed my program director. I failed the audience. I failed the chair.

My program director taught me a lesson at that moment that I have never forgotten. In fact, what he did was so powerful that I've used the example in business courses I've taught since that time. After my made-for-television screwup, he didn't fire me. Instead, he looked me squarely in the eyes and stated emphatically, "Get the hell back in there!" And with his encouragement, that was precisely what I did. I returned to the microphone and listened intently to his every direction. His faith in me helped launch a lengthy career in radio that I've cherished. It was a very special time in my life as I honed a craft that had a dramatic effect on the person I am today.

I learned a life lesson that I would not soon forget. That is, when things seem implausible, don't give up.

Certainly, there are times when charging ahead with a particular cause would not be wise. However, if it's your dream or something that absolutely needs to happen, don't give up. Not every door will swing open for you, but if the situation aligns with your hopes, dreams, and ambitions, push ahead and see what happens. It's a lesson I placed into practice as I moved into larger markets over the next few years. Ultimately, I lost my job in broadcasting due to the downturned economy but have always treasured those years behind the microphone. And the important lesson I learned from my program director those many ago has helped me stay the course through some very challenging days, even with PCS.

My brain injury had seemingly robbed me of so much, but it was a new day, and a new teaching opportunity had arrived. I had prepared my lesson plan, and Kindra was driving me to the college. It was the first day of a new term, and the college was bustling with students making their way about the campus. As a proud post-secondary institution, the college had several campuses spread throughout the area for the convenience and accommodation of a large student body. I was assigned to a campus that offered career-technical training, numerous transfer courses, and an extensive arts curriculum. I was impressed with its indoor fountains, unique study spaces, and a park for visiting or relaxing. It was an awesome campus, and I was thrilled to be back at the helm.

Kindra dropped me near a large double-door main entry. With my tote on wheels, I headed inside the building to locate my classroom. Since this was the first day of the term, I decided to show up early to make certain I understood how to operate the teacher's desk computer and overhead equipment. My previous teaching experience would come in handy while preparing to meet my new group of adult learners. I had just finished double-checking my lesson plan and the equipment when the first student walked through the doors and was soon followed by several more.

In some ways, teaching reminded me of my old job in the radio field. I loved interviewing people on my daily talk show. My in-studio guests shared their strong opinions and passions on various topics or upcoming events. I always came prepared with a list of questions but soon learned the art of extemporaneous banter. It was an excellent way to prepare for the classroom. In my first experience as a classroom teacher, I taught a course in business ethics. I worked hard at creating an environment where students felt safe to share their ideas and opinions, even if those opinions ran contrary to others. That was my skill set as an instructor, helping students feel safe, comfortable, and confident. And that was my same objective this time around—to be a cheerleader for the students as they began their very important journey in the collegiate world and beyond.

My classroom was nearly full of students as the last few made their way in. By their facial expressions, I could see they were as excited as I was. I could also tell they were nervous as they introduced themselves to one another and then finding a seat. For them, it was a different journey than mine. I didn't yet know their previous life experience, but I knew mine. I was on a path that included some unexpected twists and turns. The car accident a few months earlier seemed to derail my life for a time, but I was now ready to get things underway again. This job had provided me another opportunity to be the best version of myself and hopefully make a positive difference in the lives of others.

The wall clock moved to 8:00 a.m., and the room became quiet. My heart was beating a little faster than usual, but I had everything I needed. The overhead projector was turned to the on position. Check. My lesson plan was placed directly in front of me on the lectern. Check. Handouts were laid perfectly adjacent to the lesson plan. Check. The desk computer and mouse were at the ready. Check. It was time to take a deep breath and welcome my new class of students. I made my way out from behind the lectern and stood before about thirty adult learners, each with their own life story. My effectiveness as an instructor had always been to make my students feel as comfortable as possible, and this day would be no different. I was ready to pick up where I left off.

"Good morning, everyone," I said with a smile. The students responded in kind as they looked about the room. They were adjusting to their new environment and ready to get their college experience underway. I continued, "My name is Dr. Mike Arthur, and I am so excited to be your instructor for this course." So far, so good. No slipups, so I was ready to launch this ship! So much water had run under the bridge, and my journey had led me to this very moment in time. From this day forward, I would put the hardships behind me. It was time to, once again, teach a college course, and I was thrilled beyond belief. It was time to be an instructor who sets a positive tone and inspires excellence from his students. After a long hiatus, I had finally returned and secretly wondered if Eden might be around the next bend.

I invited my new students to introduce themselves: "Nothing too awkward, just share your name, as well as your educational and career objectives." The first bullet in my lesson plan not only provided an opportunity to get acquainted but also gave me a brief pause to collect my thoughts while the students were speaking. After all, I was concerned about my PCS and how I would perform on my first day back to work. I had prepared and designed built-in accommodations for myself. In my lesson plan, I included "escape" opportunities in case I found myself struggling with processing, speech, or some other issue. I had created a fail-safe system that required the students be highly involved throughout the class to ensure that things ran smoothly.

The sharing time went very well as they bantered and got to know one another. The class was off to a good start, and it was time for bullet number two. Once again, I opened my mouth and began to speak. However, this time, I needed to deliver longer sentences and with more detail. That's when it happened; my words escaped me and became garbled. Worry quickly turned to panic as I scrambled in my mind on what to do. Stress and anxiety were always a catalyst to increased symptoms. My prepa- ration time, complete with a detailed lesson plan, didn't help since I was drawing a complete blank. I quickly tried to cover myself, but my corrections were also unintelli- gible. Everything got quiet. I could tell my students were getting increasingly uncomfortable. One student asked if she could step out to get me a cup of water. I shook my head to say no. I tried speaking a third time, but those words were no better.

On our way to the college that morning, I experienced some minor symptoms, but with the contingency plan in place, I was feeling good about the day. My head was hurt- ing, probably around level four, with ten being the worst. The pain was in the temple regions and toward the back of my head. I was also experiencing the all-too-familiar numbness across my forehead and difficulty concentrating. I didn't worry too much since I had already completed my lesson plan. Furthermore, I had built-in escape options in case things got worse. But there was no account for the loss of speaking or the complete inability to stay focused on the current or next step. I had completely lost my ability to lead the class.

I needed to get composure, so I told the students I'd be right back and quickly exited the classroom. I spent the next few minutes pacing outside in the hallway. I walked back and forth with my head held low. I was crestfallen and had no idea what to do. This was a brand-new job, another opportunity for me. I wanted to make a positive difference for my students. I wanted to take care of my family. The interview went so well with not even one garbled word. There was excellent banter. There was confidence. They wanted me on their team. I wanted to be on their team. But there I was, out in the hallway, feeling hopeless again. I had made every contingency possible to make the new job work. Not only did it not work, it imploded in front of a live audience.

The conversation fell quickly to a hush as I reentered the classroom and made my way to the front. Still cautious about speaking, I retrieved a stack of syllabi and began to distribute them among the students. It was dead quiet and uncomfortable. There I was, an instructor who placed high importance on a comfortable environment for his students, and I was the one making it extremely awkward. After everyone received a syllabus, I gathered more handouts and distributed those as well. Now my heart was pounding even faster. I also felt a goose-bump sensation around the left side of my head. I was embarrassed, and I could feel my face begin to blush. I finished handing out the course information and sent the students home. They were first-time college students attending their first day of class, and I had to send them home.

Once the students had all gone, I sat alone on an outdoor bench, waiting for Kindra to come and get me. As usual, the Texas sun offered no sympathy whatsoever, with its glaring brightness and excessive heat. I just sat there disoriented, discouraged, and confused. What was wrong? I wondered. Why couldn't my family practitioner, or some other specialist, give me concrete answers? Should someone have warned me about the potential consequences of heading back to work too soon? How would I know when I had crossed the threshold into normalcy? Was there a quick fix to this extremely frustrating situation? Was there a pill that I could take to solve this unrelenting nightmare?

PCS doesn't play by normal rules. There's no rhyme or reason to the intensity of symptoms or length of stay. They come and go of their own volition. It's a heart-wrenching process void of any predictable pattern or common sense. When the symptoms subside, everything seems almost normal. In fact, the symptoms are so conniving; they convince you that they've gone for good after a few days of relative normalcy. Then, with the smallest level of stress or anxiety, they come back with more intensity than ever, ruling your life for the next several days to weeks.

My first supervisor in radio broadcasting had it right. One does need grit about moving forward no matter the challenge or circumstance. He was right on target, and I appreciated his wisdom. But this was a different animal. Persistent PCS and its associated symptoms don't care about your pain or agony. It's not concerned with your stumbling of words. It has one purpose, to throw your life into chaos. And to that end, it brings its contingent of soldiers to affect the whole of your life: headaches, dizziness,

fatigue, irritability, anxiety, insomnia, loss of concentration and memory, ringing in the ears, noise and light sensitivity, and word finding. Each of these brings its own
challenges, but experiencing an ensemble of the symptoms can be overwhelming.

My return to teaching turned into a fiasco as the symptoms became more pronounced. Even more problematic
than my stumbling of words was my difficulty processing information. My specific injuries had affected my
processing and short-term memory skills, two of the
most needed capabilities when leading a group of students. Back in the early days of radio, there was a hand-
held magnetic device programmers used to erase content
from a cart/tape. Once the cart/tape was erased, a new
commercial or other content could be recorded on that
same cart/tape. That is precisely how my head felt on
that first day back to work. I felt as though someone had
held the device close to my head and emptied it of all
usable content. My processing ability was nearly gone
while in front of my class.

After returning from the college, we headed out to our
favorite walking path. We found our preferred bench with
plenty of privacy and a nearby pond just a stone's toss
away. My thoughts were far away as I pondered how
much time I had put into the teaching profession, and now
it seemed to be slipping further and further from me. Kindra, always up for a meaningful conversation, was determined to forge ahead. She is an excellent communicator,
seeming to know the perfect anecdote for most conversations. However, she would have her work cut out for her
on this day since I had sunk to a new low. Meanwhile,
some nearby ducks milled playfully across the water, with
one colorful mallard swimming close to us, helping to
break the silence.

Kindra opened up about our friends who honored us with an anniversary gift after we were married for just one year. Bill and Judy were good friends and became our mentors in many ways, helping us navigate the challenges of a young marriage. Having grown up in New York, Bill had a strong personality, but he also had a heart as big as the state of Texas. We were so excited to travel with them to Maui and stayed in their timeshare for several days. It was the trip of a lifetime, and we couldn't be more thrilled. To help prepare for our grand adventure, we doubled up our exercise regimen and read everything we could about the island. Maui is a breathtaking tropical paradise where visitors are welcomed with plenty to see and do. Our temporary home in Kihei, located on Maui's southwest shore, was the sunniest and driest end of the island and beach-combing territory for the oceanfront enthusiast. It had the most awe-inspiring views we'd ever seen.

Bill and Judy suggested that we travel the famous road to Hana as "alone time" to celebrate our anniversary. The recommendation also came with Bill's caveat to be extra careful. Apparently, the road to Hana came with beautiful scenery but was also notorious for its 620 hairpin turns just to make things interesting. At the time, the road was mostly void of barriers to keep vehicles from careening down a rock cliff to the ocean below. As well, many parts of the road squeezed from two thin lanes down to one making the drive even more treacherous. Bill reminded me that it wasn't for the faint of heart and I should keep my bride safe and sound. We were so excited for the journey that we probably didn't pay enough heed to his warning as we hurried out the door.

With its cliffs cloaked in ravishing greens and valleys boastful of waterfalls, the highway gives glimpses of the ocean as it curves its way through beautiful gardens and its famous rainbow eucalyptus. It's a tropical paradise that leaves one's mind forever imprinted. Given my post-concussion symptoms, Kindra had offered the perfect metaphor that moved beyond my current reasoning power and into my deeper self. She had mulled what to say and found the analogy of a lifetime. Somehow, she gained my full attention and kept it throughout our time together out on the bench.

Kindra reminded me that the road to Hana on Maui Island was the most amazing place we'd ever been in our young marriage. The tropical paradise that envelops the road represents the pinnacle of creation. Like the Wasatch Mountains in northern Utah, the vegetation speaks a profound language with its message of hope and peace. And along the road to Hana, one comes across the Garden of Eden and Botanical Arboretum. The area is fitly named due to its native and indigenous plants and exotic flora, all set within a tropical rain forest. It's quite the site to behold. Kindra reminded me that we had come across two Eden's in our time together, one early in our marriage and the other just before the accident. Each offers its own unique form of beauty and challenges.

We talked into the evening as the sun began to set. The ducks were quiet now and perched on nearby rocks and a small embankment. We were nearly ready for home when Kindra looked directly into my eyes. "That road to Hana was treacherous." She continued, "Do you remember how narrow it was? It was a hazardous journey, but we made it. Do you recall what we found at the end, a few miles past the town of Hana? There was a glorious little church sitting there for decades. It was more than a vacation get-away—it was a message that still speaks to us today."

The pathway of life is not always easy. There are twists and turns and, sometimes, unexpected tragedies. How can inexpressible beauty coexist with indescribable danger? Much like the contrast between the winding road to Hana and the beauty that surrounds it was our experience in northern Utah. We were ecstatic about our new beginning in a land of hope and opportunity. Our stroll through the mountain town of Eden seemed to underscore that we had made the right decision by moving away from our long-time home. It was an inspired weekend, only two days before the accident. In only a matter of three seconds, the accident took our dreams and aspirations, turned them upside down, and changed everything.

The road to Hana provided an incredible contrast of light and darkness, certainty and uncertainty, hope and hopelessness, strength and fear. But Kindra asked me to recall what we had found at the end. About eight miles south of Hana was the little historic Palapala Ho'omau Church, which sat a few yards from the cliff. Not far from the church, among the lush landscape, was a granite slab laid upon lava stones. Buried on this site was the famous aviator Charles Lindbergh. I had studied this aviator when I was younger and was honored to pay my respects. There was a special solemnity about his resting place there near the palm trees. It was a wonderful surprise to stumble upon the grave of this world-renowned aviator, and we took it all in.

But there was something uniquely special not far from Lindbergh's grave. As we were admiring the awe-inspiring Pacific Ocean, we noticed a little wooden cross. Directly in front of the cliff, which dropped precipitously to the ocean below, was the little wooden cross standing no more than three feet tall. From our vantage near the gravesite, the ocean created the perfect backdrop to the symbol and gave it fanfare with its crashing waves. It was a special moment for us, but there was even more to behold. As we approached the cross to look over the cliffs, we noticed an inscribing that had the exact month, day, and year of our marriage. For us, it didn't mean the end of something but the beginning. It represented peace. It represented beauty. And it represented hope.

Kindra emphasized that the head injury had changed the trajectory of our lives, but peace, beauty, and hope were never far away. It was the same on the road to Hana; one wrong turn could lead to destruction, but a proper focus brings in the light. Find a way to incorporate optimism into your life. It's that deep and abiding place within the soul where resolve is found. When you truly accept the journey before you, even if it's the most challenging of circumstances, it's the first of many steps on your road to healing. Healing of your body, soul, and spirit. Find your resolve and settle there. Run to hope and never let go.

4

Post-Concussion Syndrome and Work

Preparing for my interview at the college took a great deal of time, but I felt ready. With hours of preparation behind me and a presentation that went better than I could have imagined, I was offered a position that same day. The interviewers seemed genuinely excited to include me as part of their team, and I was excited too. The symptoms were still recurring, but I sincerely believed I could be successful. I showed up to my new class well prepared, even designing specific accommodations in case there were problems. Unfortunately, the fail-safes didn't work, and I had to send my students home. It was one of my most difficult days, as I had to grapple with my new reality, a reality that prevented me from doing my most favorite work.

The human body is an incredibly beautiful and complex machine. When that machine's functionality is disrupted by an unexpected event, such as a TBI, the healing process can take some time. Sandra Duran fully understands the dichotomy of the pre- and post-injury brain. As someone who has always believed in the benefits of staying active, she has kicked out 140.6 miles in a swim, bike, and run event. Sadly, in September 2020, she injured her head after taking a nasty fall on her bicycle. Like most

10.4324/9781003216056-4

head-injury patients, the journey has not been easy, but she tries to stay optimistic. From deep within her soul, Sandra wrote a poem that speaks to the raw emotion of living life with PCS:

> I miss my brain.
> I miss my brain before it smacked the hard, unforgiving
>   concrete nestled inside my bicycle helmet.
> I miss my brain when it could take me on a 15-mile
>   trail run or 20-mile hike and be perfectly OK.
> I miss my brain when EVERYTHING was easier.
> I miss my brain when coordinating activities at work
>   was second nature.
> I miss my brain when it remembered basic stuff like
>   what it was doing the moment it was doing it.
> I miss my brain when it didn't hurt EVERY single day.
> I miss my brain when it wasn't injured.
> Why couldn't I have just broken my arm?
> I love life too much for this crap.
> I miss my brain.

Sandra concluded, "Although I am not yet healed from my concussion . . . I am slowly making improvements. Little did I know concussions take lots of time if you don't allow your brain the time needed to heal. My balance and equilibrium are all out of whack, and running literally rattles my brain, causing dizziness, head pressure, and fatigue. You just end up feeling miserable and then depressed. You can't do what you so love to do. So I have found other things to maintain my fitness, but walking has become such a blessing. The little things appear that may have otherwise been just a blur as you whizzed past on your morning 14-mile run."

Sandra perfectly described life for the person who struggles with a head injury. It's not an easy path, but if one allows, the little things will begin to illumine, bringing about a heightened awareness of the environment and a new level of appreciation. It's about love over loneliness. Hope over hopelessness. It's about embracing the light over the darkness and being determined not to let the depression win. One of the most challenging aspects of PCS is the negative feelings and emotions that come with a brain that isn't quite healed yet. It's overwhelming at times. If you're not having this sort of issue, you are fortunate as these are common symptoms. Also, in ancillary circumstances, such as an unsupportive employer or loss of work, the negative feelings move in like a flood.

I haven't yet been able to work full-time, and it has been an emotional battle. But it's a battle that I'm winning, and you can too. Recognize what you can do, and then do those things to the best of your ability. As well, understand your limitations and live within that sphere until you are able to take on new challenges and meet new goals. I am convinced that it's in your mind, deep within your most imaginative self, that healing can take root. What is it that draws the creative juices from you? What are you most excited about that requires a deeper level within your brain? Scientists have discovered that our brains have incredible potential, even to the trillions of synaptic connections. What will your new connections be? What draws you out of your routine and lifts you to new places in your imagination?

The human brain is as vast as the cosmos and equally as intriguing. Let your brain take you to new heights beyond the stars, and don't let the depression win. You still have great value. Look for wonderment. Though everyone is unique, I've found my greatest creative imagination out in nature. Before my accident, I was awe-inspired by the wonder of the Wasatch Mountains. After my accident, I remained the same. My brain injury did not affect my willingness, desire, and ability to recognize nature's voice. If you'll listen, you can hear it too. Allow yourself to hear the whispers of nature. The tiniest little breeze can prod your imagination sparking your synapses and nudging you to wholeness. Allow your imagination to carry you to that place Lindbergh treasured as "the remotest part of the sea."

You truly are running a *marathon* and not a sprint. This will take some time. You'll have difficult days, even some dark days but don't let that rule over you. Accept and know that better days will come; they always do. Never let the darkness win over your creative, imaginative, and hopeful self. If you lack support from your immediate family, work, and/or friends, find support. For the brain-injured person with PCS, there are specialists that truly care and will support you. Don't be afraid to reach out. Build your circle of light and march forward. Living with the realities of PCS and its symptoms is not easy, but you can reign victorious. Search answers in every corner of your life, including your vocation, whatever that might be.

Every career has its own challenges that can affect how an employee with PCS is able to function. Imagine, for example, if a police officer sustained a head injury after chasing someone trying to get away. Police officers have a huge responsibility in protecting lives and property and by enforcing laws and regulations. They respond to emergencies that require good judgment and processing skills. They conduct on-scene interviews, arrest and process criminals, testify in court, and need to have the ability to use proper judgment on when and how to use force. If a police officer has PCS symptoms, such as memory problems and trouble concentrating, how would they do their job well? Further, how might a case be affected if the officer couldn't recall the description of the suspect or any unusual circumstances related to a specific scene?

What about the pharmacist with PCS? Doing the work of a pharmacist can be extremely challenging throughout an entire workday. Among their many responsibilities, they dispense medications to patients and medical facilities. Their knowledge of chemistry, not to mention an in-depth understanding of anatomy and physiology, is detrimental to their daily performance. Most pharmacies stay extremely busy from the time they open in the morning until they lock the doors late at night. The pharmacist suffering from PCS would struggle to stay on task, trying to maintain a high standard of care. As with other critical jobs, mistakes could be devastating for the patients they serve.

Whether you're employed as a police officer, pharmacist, physician, paramedic, accountant, millworker, service industry worker, or some other valued position, every job has its challenges. When I worked in radio broadcasting, I provided both recorded and live news for five radio stations. Each and every second of the day was accounted for. It was a bit like juggling plates on sticks in front of a live audience. There was no room for error since the result would be dead air. Dead air is a huge misstep in radio since it's unprofessional and can ultimately affect the bottom line and listenership. I am quite certain that if I had gotten my brain injury while working in broadcasting, I would have quit or been fired within a very short period of time.

Although TBI and PCS have been highlighted in the news in recent years, it's important to note that many employers are still not up-to-date on the latest research related to employees with head injuries. In fact, the prevailing logic remains that if football players are able to sustain repeated concussions and get back to work, certainly an employee with one or two concussions could do the same. It's important that employers be up on the possible health implications of PCS and that they understand the potential costs associated with treatment as well. In fact, TBI is connected to high healthcare costs, both for individuals and society.

Out of concern for the health and welfare of the employees and the potential costs incurred for treatment, the employer should recognize the common symptoms of concussion and PCS:

- Headaches
- Irritability
- Nausea
- Vomiting
- Balance and visual problems
- Dizziness
- Fatigue
- Sensitivity to noise and light
- Tingling and numbness
- Ringing in the ears

Workers may report the following:

- Feeling mentally foggy or slowed down
- Having difficulty concentrating
- Being forgetful or confused

Also, employees might experience anxiety, blurry vision, insomnia, and sometimes, decreases in taste and smell. An employer might also notice that an employee takes more time than usual to answer questions and might ask that questions be repeated. They might also seem emotional and tired from a lack of sleep.

When you return to work after injuring your brain, it can be an uphill battle that is hard to win. Your work ethic hasn't changed. Your desire for excellence is still intact. You're the same person you were before the accident, but now you've got a brain injury that affects your cognitive abilities. PCS is a quiet reality that doesn't bust into a room demanding everyone's attention. It's an invisible injury that reduces one's previous abilities limiting one's effectiveness on the jobsite. Simple everyday tasks can be forgotten. If there are more complex requirements, those, too, can be fumbled, creating a work environment that is unsustainable. Add that to your inability to perform at your previous high level, and the *invisible* component of your injury might cause your supervisor to question your loyalty.

If PCS symptoms are difficult for family members to comprehend, imagine how a supervisor must feel. From their perspective, you don't seem much different from before your accident. Same voice. Same smile. Same walk. Same you. So what's the problem? Just keep doing those things you did before the accident and everything will be just fine. Herein lies the problem for significant people in your life; they can't see inside your brain. They don't understand that you're not processing information like you used to. They are not grasping that, perhaps, your short-term memory has been affected, and you might not recall important information as you once did. From the outside perspective, you seem normal, but you're falling short in your work life.

What is it about PCS that can cause angst in the employer-employee relationship? Sure, there are employers who've been trained on post-concussion symptoms and have genuine concern for the well-being of the workers.

But based on testimonies shared via online support groups, some employees with PCS experience nightmarish scenarios with their managers. Managers don't always get it. Many don't understand the implications of PCS, nor do they wish to. Their primary goal is a productive department, come hell or high water. If you're no longer able to perform at your best, then "don't let the door hit you on the way out" can be the mindset. This scenario is far too common and shouldn't be. For supervisors willing to learn about the illness for the betterment of their organization, good research is available.

With an eye toward the informal qualitative approach to research, I've gathered a sampling of comments made by people I've met who have been diagnosed with PCS. In the process, I looked for common statements, or themes, that indicated a problem in the employee-employer relationship. The comments are paraphrased below without compromising original meaning:

1. "My supervisor has informed me that I can't return to work until I am able and without any type of accommodations."
2. "I've always had a good relationship with my boss. That is, until after my head injury and PCS. Things are really weird between us now. I'm afraid I might be a short-timer."
3. "I don't feel like myself anymore. Work has been especially challenging. I had to explain my PCS and how it can affect my productivity. My boss seemed disinterested and like he didn't believe me. I need to figure something out before I get fired."

Of course, many supervisors fully support their workers when they have personal or medical issues that prevent them from performing at their best. However, for employees who do not get that type of support, the work environment can become a catalyst to increasing symptoms through anxiety and depression. In my experience with PCS, I've found that stress and anxiety become precursors to increased severity of symptoms, such as headaches, memory loss, and difficulty concentrating. Herein lies one of the many challenges for the employee with PCS. The lack of support by a supervisor can actually increase symptoms making work tasks that much more difficult. For those employers who display genuine empathy and understand the reality of PCS and the repercussions of its symptoms, below are suggested accommodations that can provide realistic goals for the employee:

- Provide a schedule that reduces total hours worked within a given day and week.
- Provide additional breaks. If possible, allow the employee some alone time in a quiet room without lights or distractions.
- Restructure the employee's job responsibilities. This might entail temporarily reassigning the more complicated job tasks to another employee.
- Ask that the employee write things down. Making lists early in the workday before the employees' brain gets tired might help alleviate confusion and disorientation later in the shift.
- Incorporate electronic scheduling apps if that helps.
- Provide additional support unique to the struggles of your employee.

Providing accommodations is a good place to start for the employee who is actually able to stay somewhat focused.

Unfortunately, returning to full-time work is not an option for every person who sustains a head injury. Other than recognizing certain characteristics, such as mechanism of injury, previous head injury, and/or other standard diagnostic mechanisms, determining a reliable prognosis is not always straightforward. Certainly, your healthcare provider can make estimates based on similar cases or previous experience, but the process is challenging. In my case, I have been able to work part-time since my accident, but full-time employment is not yet on the horizon. I feel fortunate to have found an excellent physiatrist at UT Southwestern Medical Center in the United States. He has directed and supported me along the way, closely following a holistic approach. It's from that vantage that I've undergone extensive testing and treatment at an excellent neurological clinic. As part of an outpatient rehabilitation program, I was assigned to the clinic three days per week and several hours per day. The sessions mostly focused on occupational therapy, psychological therapy, physical therapy, and speech therapy. I was also given an extensive battery of tests as a way to recognize improvement throughout the treatment.

Neurological clinics provide a team of healthcare professionals who are experts in their respective fields. The goal for patients is that they feel at home and, sometimes, even taking lunch breaks with members of the technician team and other patients. I did feel welcome from the first day and committed myself wholly to the process. It was a nice facility with a large lunchroom centrally located. The experience was akin to attending classes, one after the other, at a local college or high school. However, the sessions were not a cakewalk as the technicians worked hard with the best possible outcomes in mind. There was no standing around or wasting time. Even my physical therapy sessions were exhausting and required a level of stamina to complete the therapy requirements.

Neurological clinics help determine functionality and provide support for both body and brain. In my case, extensive testing revealed a deficit in my executive functioning capabilities, as well as processing and short-term memory. I was given a battery of tests for an evaluation of speech, language, and cognitive functioning skills. Among the tests were the Repeatable Battery for Assessment of Neuropsychological Status (RBANS), a speech-language screening, and the Functional Assessment of Verbal Reasoning and Executive Skills (FAVRES). Results from the FAVRES indicated I had sustained deficits in the speed of processing, memory, and semantic fluency. RBANS, in particular, showed severe deficits in both immediate and delayed memory. The test also indicated problems with the speed of processing, memory, and semantic fluency.

Having a better understanding of your functionality is an important place to begin. The clarity provided by extensive testing not only provides specialists with a direction for treatment, it helps give the head-injured patient a better grasp on their condition and what lies ahead. My speech therapist was extraordinary in her ability to explain the results in a kind, empathetic, and professional manner, but I felt overwhelmed with the process. I tried my best on each test, and the outcome still showed significant deficits in several key areas. Hiding how I really felt inside as the therapist explained the results was not easy. At the moment, I actually felt like a shell of my former self. It was an uncomfortable experience, but it was something I needed to hear and an important step in my road to recovery both in my personal and work life.

Like many head-injured patients, I have often struggled with feelings of despair since the accident but have determined to continue with the neurological treatments and, at some point, find myself again. Daniel Siegel, a clinical professor of psychiatry, stated, "Internal mental experience is not the product of a photographic process. Internal reality is in fact constructed by the brain as it interacts with the environment in the present, in the context of its past experiences and expectancies of the future. At the level of perceptual categorizations, we have reached a land of mental representations quite distant from the layers of the world just inches away from their place inside the skull. This is the reason why each of us experiences a unique way of minding the world" (Siegel, 2020, pp. 166–167).

My specialized treatment, along with the passing of time, encouraged improved processing ability and a higher level of functionality. However, my circumstance is unique to me and does not necessarily represent the challenges of other patients who suffer from a head injury. There are different types of head injuries affecting different parts of their brain. Also, jobs have unique intellectual requirements complicating a surefooted prognosis. Certainly, brain-injured patients fall into one of three categories related to their work capabilities: those who can return to work full-time, those who can only work part-time, and those who can't work at all. In my current situation, I still fall into the "part-time" category.

Along with my previous job as vice principal, I taught one course for a university before my accident and still teach that same course today. I've found that my post-concussion symptoms wane in their intensity, which has allowed me to work when I am able. I communicate with students, grade assignments, comment on the discussion boards, and do other tasks as required. The work is asynchronous, meaning I complete the duties when I am thinking more clearly. The fact is, I still struggle with PCS symptoms. It's a strange reality that prevents me from teaching an in-class course, which is my most treasured work and ultimate goal. The head-injured person should have a goal that drives them throughout the healing process. For me, I'll know when I'm back to my old self when I can, once again, stand behind a lectern.

Returning to full-time employment should be on the radar, if possible. Given that each accident is unique, accurately predicting when someone might return to work can be a complicated process. The following characteristics play a significant role in when and how an employee might be able to return:

• Mechanism of injury
• Whether there was a previous head injury
• Presence of post-traumatic stress disorder
• Age of the patient
• Physical condition of the patient
• Psychological condition of the patient
• Social health of the patient

Mechanism of Injury

The mechanism of injury is the manner in which a physical injury took place. The injury could have happened from a fall of some sort, a motor vehicle accident, or any number of other circumstances leading to a head injury. Mechanism of injury is a complex term used to help medical professionals determine the potential severity of damage to a person's body in relation to fractures, internal organ damage, and even wounding.

Whether There Was a Previous Head Injury

Incurring a second head injury within a given amount of time can be very troublesome. Second impact syndrome

(SIS), as it's called, happens when the brain swells rapidly shortly after a person suffers a second concussion before symptoms from an earlier concussion have subsided. This event is rare, but when it does happen, it can oftentimes be fatal.

Presence of Post-Traumatic Stress Disorder

According to the Mental Health Foundation, post-traumatic stress disorder (PTSD) is "a condition that can develop after exposure to extremely stressful and traumatizing events. People experiencing PTSD may have symptoms such as flashbacks or panic attacks." The condition is often found in head-injured patients and can be problematic both in treatment and functionality.

Age of the Patient

In their research, Gardner et al. (2018) point out that "on average, older adults with TBI have higher mortality, slower rates of functional and cognitive recovery, and worse functional outcomes post-TBI compared to their younger counterparts." Although some researchers argue there is unlikely to be an older age range where outcomes become quite noticeably worse, other researchers have found an "inflection point in the fourth of fifth decade of life."

Physical Condition of the Patient

Research is readily available on the benefits of routine exercise on physical and cognitive health. In their study, Gomes-Osman et al. found that exercise is associated with improved cognitive performance, with or without cognitive impairment. The researchers state, "The assessment of the relationship between improved cognition and various measures of exercise dose (session duration, weekly minutes, frequency, total weeks, and total hours) revealed a significant correlation with total hours. Improvements in global cognition, processing speed/attention, and executive function were most stable and consistent."

Psychological and Social Health of the Patient

The psychological and social health of the patient both play significant factors regarding recovery and whether one can return to work given a specific period of time.

One way to determine if you're ready to take on more work is to simply test the waters. Teaching one course online has worked out very well for me simply because the course is asynchronous, so I can work when my symptoms are less troublesome. I do struggle if my symptoms are ongoing for several days but the intensity level on a given day seems to wane as well. The course has been a godsend and has also helped me to exercise my brain in my ongoing effort for better functionality. As well, writing outside the graduate course has worked out in a similar fashion. I primarily do the work when I am able to think clearly without too much pain, discomfort, or distraction. If you suffer from PCS and want to increase your work hours, whether you're increasing from zero or a part-time situation, talk with your doctor to see if they green light the idea. If he or she believes it's worth a try, consider talking with your supervisor about an incremental approach.

Below is a straightforward plan that can be adjusted based on your specific brain injury and work-related profile. It's a rule-of-thumb approach, not necessarily research-based, but follows a 10% rule (PCS 10% Rule) for increasing work hours:

Example 1

Currently working: 10 hours per week
Add: One hour per week for two weeks (10%)
Symptom Results: If at the end of week two your symptoms did not increase, try adding two to three additional hours for weeks three and four. If at the end of week four your symptoms did not increase, try adding more hours as you feel comfortable. At this point, it's trial and error. Try to find a range of hours that works for you specifically in your recovery process.

Example 2

Currently working: 20 hours per week
Add: Two hours per week for two weeks
Symptom Results: If at the end of week two your symptoms did not increase, try adding three to four additional hours for weeks three and four. If at the end of week four your symptoms did not increase, try adding more hours as you feel comfortable. At this point, it's trial and error. Try to find a range of hours that works for you specifically in your recovery process.

Whether you're *not working at all* and want to return, or you're *currently working part-time* and hope to increase those hours, a common-sense approach is best. Just remember, if you're currently not working, you might discover that you're still unable to work. If you are working part-time and want to increase your hours, you might learn that having more hours is not yet feasible. The PCS 10% Rule provides a game plan for both you and your employer to determine your current capabilities. Once again, your doctor will need to agree that a plan like this is right for your situation. Also, be aware that even if you discover that you are not yet ready for increased work hours, you can try following a plan like this again in a few months. However, for some patients suffering from persistent PCS symptoms, returning to work may never be an option. The idea here is that you incorporate a plan that provides answers regarding your capabilities.

As someone who has endured ongoing symptoms of PCS, lasting longer than three years, I believe the PCS 10% Rule is appropriate for determining one's capabilities related to time at work. One of the major symptoms of PCS is that the brain gets tired or foggy quite readily. In my situation, if my symptoms last several days or even weeks, I can't even drive for more than one to two hours during an entire day. Should this be a rule of thumb for all patients with PCS? Of course not. Adding to the complexity of the human brain, the type of injuries sustained, and individual characteristics, every patient needs to know what their specific limitations are (sometimes through trial-and-error). The PCS 10% Rule takes a conservative approach since injured brains can tire easily.

Once an injured brain gets tired or foggy, there is a dramatic effect on its ability to process, which makes working at a jobsite, or any other location for that matter, very difficult. If your production levels are adequate, and you are not having increased symptoms with your current work schedule and level of responsibility, ask your doctor and supervisor about applying the PCS 10% Rule. After incorporating the approach into your work schedule, you might discover that you aren't able to increase your hours at this time.

For some patients with PCS, increasing work hours and responsibilities is not only possible; it's a good thing to do. The PCS 10% Rule takes into account the seriousness of your brain injury and gently increases your work schedule to provide a baseline on functionality. Certainly, if you're already struggling with symptoms at work, this plan is not right for you. However, if symptoms have been minimal, and they continue to be minimal two weeks after initiating the PCS 10% Rule, try adding even more hours than recommended. The idea at this point is to use your common sense so you don't become overburdened with symptoms possibly causing an injury or worse.

In addition to the PCS 10% Rule, consider changing up your work responsibilities. This process is somewhat of a balancing act and should run in cohort with your adjusted hours. In other words, if your supervisor is willing, try adjusting your work schedule and responsibilities at the same time. You might discover a happy medium that works well as you continue to increase both your hours and duties. There are many ways to adjust your schedule and work responsibilities to accommodate your symptoms with an eye on getting back to normal, if possible. If you haven't been able to work at all since your accident, and you believe you might be ready, try working two to three days per week to start. Return with shorter hours and take more breaks throughout the day. Also, return with less of a workload and consider taking on a different, less demanding role if that will help.

If you have seen improvement in the PCS symptoms, and the objective is returning to work full-time at some point, this is an admirable goal. A UK-based organization called Headway: The Brain Injury Association, offers six strategies for getting back to work after a brain injury.

According to Headway, "With the right support and planning, many people do successfully get back to work after brain injury." The following are the six strategies that Headway provides that can help you in the process:

Seek Support

It is important to choose a job that is right for you; even though you will likely know best about your personal skills, interests, and experience, it can be very useful to seek advice and support from family, close friends, and professional services. This can be particularly helpful if you experience memory issues, difficulties with making decisions, or reduced self-awareness. Remember that accepting help from others is a sign of strength, not weakness, and the right support can make a successful return to work much easier.

Only Return When You Are Ready

One of the most common problems brain injury survivors face when returning to work is that they return too soon because they do not realize how the effects of their brain injury will impact their work performance. This is a particular problem when a good physical recovery has been made, as people often assume that cognitive abilities have also recovered. Returning to work often reveals the full extent of difficulties, and returning too soon can damage confidence if performance doesn't meet expectations. It is advisable to avoid making major decisions and becoming involved in stressful situations until you feel you are ready. This is especially the case in jobs with high levels of stress and pressure and where margins for error are small. Mistakes made because of the injury could damage your confidence and hinder recovery. Be honest with yourself, prepare as much as possible, and don't try to rush your recovery. Remember, try not to take overtime shift work or new responsibilities until you feel ready.

Be Positive but Realistic

The attitude you have toward returning to work is very important. Research has shown that the following factors are particularly influential:

- Willingness to accept and act on honest feedback from others
- Realistic awareness and insight
- Willingness to use strategies to help with these problems
- Willingness to tell others what you need

Thinking positively does not just mean saying, "I will go back to work," but rather it means carefully considering and planning the best options. It means asking yourself, "What can I do?" "What am I going to have difficulty with?" and "How do I manage the problems?"

There is a balance to be found between positivity and realism. Unrealistic expectations can lead to disappointment and loss of self-esteem, and it is very important to think carefully about the effects of the injury and their impact on your abilities. However, it is equally important to be positive and committed to the path you choose to follow.

Communicate with Your Employer

You do not have a legal duty to disclose your brain injury to an employer, and they are not allowed to ask questions about your health unless it is directly related to the job requirements. However, you should always disclose information related to your health if it may put yourself or other people at risk. The following suggestions can help to ensure that you are keeping communication open with your employer:

- Make sure you keep in fairly regular contact with your employer while you are away. You might wish to ask a family member or a friend to do this for you if it is difficult to keep contact yourself.
- Make sure you understand your sick pay entitlement, and do not be afraid of discussing this with your employer.
- Provide your employer with information about brain injury, such as other Headway publications. Of particular relevance is the Headway factsheet.

Adaptations to the workplace—a guide for employers:

- If you have a DEA or a relevant healthcare professional, ask if they would be willing to talk to your employer.
- Be honest with your employer about your abilities. If you are unsure about your ability to complete a task, tell them.
- Make sure your employer is aware of any legal issues, such as if you have been told that you cannot drive due to an increased risk of epilepsy. This may also mean that you need to take other precautions at work.

Communicate with Your Colleagues

Again, it is up to you whether you tell colleagues about your brain injury and its effects. If you are returning to your previous job, then they will know you have been away, so it can be better to tell them something about the situation. Don't feel that you have to share anything you aren't comfortable with, but it will help people to understand and make some allowances if you are as honest as possible. The following suggestions are worth considering:

- Discuss with your employer whether you want your colleagues to know about your brain injury and any resulting disabilities. You are within your rights to ask for others not to be informed.
- Keep in touch with friends at work while you are away in order to keep them informed about the situation. If you wish, ask them to keep other colleagues up-to-date and to discretely let them know of some of the difficulties you may experience when you return.
- If starting a new job, you might like to arrange to visit your new colleagues before you formally start. It might be possible to arrange an induction process where you can discuss the situation and make sure people are aware in advance of any special arrangements.

Practice a Structured Home Program

It is important to be as prepared as possible before returning to work. An effective way of doing this is to follow a program to assess and develop the skills that will be required.

The aim is to be able to mimic a working week, so try to follow your program throughout regular working hours. Try to do this for at least two weeks before returning to work.

Some suggestions for a structured home program are as follows:

- Practice working at a computer and concentrating for as long as you will need to at work.

- Try to get up and go to bed at the times you will need to when you go back to work.
- Practice being physically active for as long as you would need to at work. This can involve any activities you like, such as mowing the lawn, shopping, cleaning the house, or exercising at the gym.

Unfortunately, not everyone dealing with PCS will be able to return, and some people might have to work under modified part-time conditions.

As you are fine-tuning your work schedule and responsibilities, be sure to maintain ongoing communication with your supervisor and any other person/department that might be important. Your path to healing from PCS is unique and should follow a well-reasoned approach that makes sense for you and your specific situation. Of course, as stated previously, not all supervisors and managers understand the implications of PCS and its symptoms. If your supervisor is reasonable, ask if they are willing to consider the latest research on the subject. The fact is, according to the *Journal of Neurosurgery*, TBI is a *silent epidemic* and affects 69 million individuals each year around the world. There is plentiful research available, which can provide important information for employees and their supervisors.

5

Post-Concussion Syndrome and Family

Perhaps no other emotional experience is as special as falling in love. Love is a complex matter that goes beyond a simple feeling or something that originates in the primitive part of the brain. It's a bonding that moves into the indescribable. Love is something more than an abstract reality. And when the trials of life move in like the waves of an ocean, love is patient and kind. Relationships are not easy, and when times get hard, as when a family member suffers from PCS it will require all the love one can muster. When your loved one has sustained a brain injury, and they forget details about an important conversation, be patient. If they break an ornate dish that has been in the family for years, be kind. If they are irritable and can't hold their tongue, be long-suffering. This does not mean that one should accept abusive behavior by another—on the contrary. But short of crossing clear lines of respect, it does mean that you're in it for the long haul. That's what love is. It's supporting one another through the various stages and circumstances of life.

When I was attending junior high school, my buddy and I decided to take a hike up a nearby mountain not far from my home. Daren Strong turned out to be a lifelong friend and an unofficial "brother" in my family. This was our first journey up this side of the mountain and would require

10.4324/9781003216056-5

that we dress in extra clothing just to stay warm. The local meteorologist had predicted a cold front with low-lying clouds and foggy conditions. The weather didn't deter our excitement for the hike and prompted us to bring along extra provisions in our backpacks. We even took along packaged military food to round out our highly anticipated journey to the unknown.

As middle-aged teens, our adventure to the top of the mountain was more than a routine hike up steep terrain. It would be a final frontier with prognostications about what we might find in the great unknown. Of the two of us, Daren was the pragmatic one; I was the dreamer. For me, our hikes represented so much more than exercise and time in the great outdoors. It was an opportunity to get my creative juices flowing, to dream about the future and its myriad of possibilities. It was where I could first hear the mountains speak but didn't yet understand their language. However, I never really fully understood nature's voice until after my accident several years later.

Our backpacks were heavy, but we were determined to keep moving up the mountain. It was bone-chilling cold, and we could see our breath as we walked along. The fog was getting thicker, but there was no conversation about turning back as we pressed harder and harder toward the summit. Eventually, we lost our bearing in the misty fog and started to doubt if we could actually make it to the summit. "Do you think we should start heading down the mountain, Daren?" He didn't say a word but pointed to a glimmer of light that was just now shining through the thick layer of clouds. He was right; we were almost free of the fog, so we pushed with even more determination and found an incredible surprise waiting for us at the top.

The sun glistened as far as our eyes could see. Below the clear blue sky was a billow of clouds that covered our hometown. It was the softest layer of clouds we'd ever seen completely hiding the thousands of homes immediately below. Just to the outer edges of the cottony billows of white were the tips of mountains surrounding in a horseshoe formation. We were in complete awe of nature's stunning display. From our vantage, there wasn't a cloud in the sky. It was peaceful, quiet, and serene. It was so bright and beautiful that we stood silent for a few minutes, just taking it all in. It was one of those extraordinary moments one remembers for a lifetime.

When the symptoms of PCS move in, it's an intense experience that sets in like a cold and damp fog confusing its victim. The peace and serenity that might have been are now gone. Also removed is the ability to process information with the same level of accuracy. It is an oppressive experience that is difficult to explain and varies from one person to the next. In my experience with PCS, the symptoms have been unreliable in their intensity and length of stay. However, after the headaches, pressure, and "brain fog" subside, there is often a ray of light like Daren spotted near the mountaintop.

Traveling is difficult but sometimes necessary for people living with a brain injury. On one important journey, I flew over 1,500 miles, which became an all-day ordeal, including travel time, layovers, and changing of flights. One of my brothers had passed away, so I was attending a special gathering for him and spending time with family. My brother's daughter did beautiful work preparing for the event, which took place in a wide-open grassy expanse complete with band shell and plenty of food. It was a special and memorable day celebrating my brother's life and his influence on each of us. But the emotional toll of grieving his loss, and the basic requirements of long-distance travel, sent my symptoms into overdrive.

Since the event was so well attended, I do not believe anyone noticed me struggling to find my words or that I was feeling disoriented. That is, with the exception of my mother. Moms always know. On this trip, I was staying in her home so hiding the symptoms wouldn't be easy. She noticed that I was withdrawn and not my normal talkative self. She also noticed how much I was struggling just to string some coherent words together. I wasn't tripping over my words with every sentence, but I did, nonetheless, struggle with normal conversation. And when symptoms are more severe, as they were during much of this trip, basic everyday routines can be fumbled or forgotten altogether. That's exactly what happened when my younger brother, Dan, showed up a few days later. My aloofness left him with very little sleep while staying at Mom's house.

The daytime temperatures were hot, with not much relief overnight. My mom bought her 1950s home in the late seventies without any sort of central air-conditioning system. Even today, the only cooling system in the entire house consists of a wall unit mounted in the family room. This means that the two guest rooms are usually hot and sultry during much of the summertime. I was staying in the north bedroom and had my things arranged for the entire visit. I have discovered since my accident that if I over-organize my life, there is less chance that I will forget something important. However, when my brother showed up, he asked if I would move to the other bedroom so he could stay in his old room.

I moved to the other room and carefully reorganized my belongings. As expected, it was exceptionally hot overnight, but I slept deep and sound. The bed was comfortable, the air was circulating, and life was good. In fact, I was so rested, it took a few minutes to crawl out of bed, get a good stretch, and head to the main area of the home. Mom was already up and offering breakfast.

"Good morning. I hope you had a good night of sleep," she said with a smile.

"Honestly, I don't think I've slept that well in a very long time," I responded.

It was about that time that Dan entered, looking like death warmed over. He was exhausted from being awake, tossing and turning most of the night. He had bags under his eyes and a voice to match.

"Dude, what happened to you?" I asked him.

Dan's usual enthusiastic personality was nowhere to be found. I didn't realize until months later that I was the one responsible for his overnight struggle because of my absentmindedness. Apparently, when I moved to the other bedroom, I took the fan with me. The result—I slept with two giant fans in my room, Dan slept with none. Looking back at what happened, we've all had a good laugh, but it's a prime example of what can happen when you're not processing information as you used to. Mom pointed out that I would never do something like that on purpose, and I wouldn't. However, overlooking common everyday steps can be a real issue for the head-injured person.

The ordeal with Dan was a one-time event that kept him from getting a good night's sleep. Imagine what it must be like for a person living full-time with someone who suffers from PCS, such as a spouse? The forgetfulness, irritability, anxiety, depression, headaches and pressure, and all the other symptoms are the fabric of an ongoing story unfolding week after week and month after month. It is a complex circumstance that requires true allegiance to the age-old vows: "for better or worse, for richer or poorer, in sickness and in health, to love and to cherish, till death do us part." Though not possible for everyone, I am thankful my partner decided she would remain true to our commitment, even through the most challenging of days.

I had been single for a few years when Kindra entered my life. At the time, I had no thought of committing to a relationship and was not necessarily looking for a partner with whom to spend my days. My main objective back then was simply to work hard, pay my bills, and take an occasional vacation. I had grandeur thoughts of visiting places like Venice, London, Rome, New Zealand and Paris. Truth be told, my traveling list was much longer, but I was determined to visit each place, even if that goal took me the next twenty years of my life. That is, until I laid my eyes on Kindra for the first time. It's hard to explain what came over me that day, but the feeling definitely lends credence to the love-at-first-sight argument.

I worked on the dry-end side of our local plywood mill and operated a Raimann machine used to replace knotholes with oval-shaped pieces of wood. The work was repetitive, requiring that I plug thousands of knotholes out of thin sheets of veneer. It was a daily task that required a great deal of accuracy and patience. Kindra was a new hire and just completing her overnight training on my machine. I noticed her immediately and was taken aback by her great big smile, bubbly personality, and the way she carried herself. I had completely forgotten that I was in the confines of a noisy plywood mill complete with band saws, lathes, lift trucks, and a host of other ear-piercing machines. For me, the room had gone quiet. There was something very special about this new employee with her lively disposition, and I wanted to learn more straight away.

I devised a simple plan—arrive a few minutes early the very next morning and ask Kindra out on a date. I remember being so nervous, I couldn't quite get the words right. "We should go out sometime," was all I could muster. She seemed pleasantly surprised, but since I hadn't offered an invitation she could accept or deny, she quickly changed the subject. On the next day, I was even more determined but still extremely nervous. Once again, there was no official invitation when I abruptly stated, "Sure would be nice to get together some time." Not surprisingly, she changed the subject once again. I was more determined than ever on the third morning. My heart was pounding as I approached the workstation early that morning, but this time, I didn't have to say a word.

She reached into her pocket and handed me a small folded piece of paper. She looked directly into my eyes and said, "That's my information. Pick me up tomorrow night at seven sharp."

If it's at all possible to fall in love on a first date, I did. My nerves completely melted away as we were enmeshed in each other's company throughout an evening filled with conversation and laughter. I don't think we ever took our eyes off one another as we enjoyed a candlelight dinner and strolled a nearby park filled with duck ponds, towering trees, flowers, and an occasional bench overlooking a fast-flowing stream with miniature boulders and crashing water. Not far from the park, we found a chocolatier offering caramel apples, fudge, and gourmet chocolates. We ordered caramel apples and strolled through the tiny town. It was the perfect last stop on a date that would launch a loving relationship for many years to come.

By no means has our life together been picture-perfect as it was on that first date. Like any other couple, we've had our struggles, but no adversity has challenged us quite like the brain injury. However, for couples (or anyone else within the family context), there is always a reason for hope. Research is available that demonstrates many mild TBI patients can improve over time. And for those individuals who continue to suffer from persistent symptoms, communication can be improved given certain criteria. Behn et al. (2019) speak about this in their research: "Communication problems are common and pervasive following [acquired brain injury] and can have a significant impact on a person's life. Setting individualized person-centered goals to address these problems is considered an important aspect of the rehabilitation process" (p. 828).

In our journey, we haven't yet made it back to Eden, but we're on our way. There are glimmers of hope shining from one month to the next. We haven't won the war, but we're making strides, and you can too. Even the day-to-day hardships can bring about their own lessons and opportunities for growth. One life lesson for me happened after I was finally able to see how my behaviors affected my wife's own emotional well-being. I didn't know to what extent until I noticed her in tears one evening. Finding her that way broke my heart. This was the same person whom I fell in love with almost from the first time I met her. Even long after we were married, her kind disposition continued shining through. But now, there she was, sitting all alone in the darkness with tears running down her face. There was no music playing as she sat on the floor with her legs crossed and hair covering most of her face. And the reality was, her pain was a direct result of my on-and-off symptoms that brought her to this place.

In the heart of the head-injured person, there might be strong love for a spouse or significant other but properly demonstrating that love can be misinterpreted during a period of intense symptoms. Conversely, for the person in the relationship without a head injury, any lack of deep and meaningful communication might make the relationship feel distant and cold. It's a complex problem that often requires the help of a counselor with a solid background in TBIs. Although there are many possibilities for potential disconnect within a relationship, here are a few examples:

- The head-injured partner is experiencing level six or higher symptoms and is having difficulty processing information and staying engaged.
   o This scenario can be interpreted as simply not caring by the non-injured significant other.
- The head-injured partner is experiencing fatigue.
   o This might be construed as a lack of interest.
- The head-injured partner is irritable.
   o This might be interpreted as dislike.

The examples above only represent a small portion of challenging scenarios that can take place within the context of a spousal or significant-other-type relationship. PCS symptoms following a TBI can even play havoc on a couple that has been together for many years.

In one study, researchers looked at marital stability after brain injury and found that 85% of survivors remained married at the two years following injury (Kreutzer et al., 2010), but other studies have shown lower survival rates. So much of what is important to the health of an intimate relationship is affected after a brain injury. Healthy marriages/ partnerships require an ongoing deep-level commitment at all levels, including communication. Unfortunately, that *access* can be severely limited when specific PCS arise, such as irritability, anxiety, and depression. Additionally, if there is an inability to process information, barriers arise, affecting the deeper mental, emotional, and physical needs of the relationship.

After seeing my wife in tears that evening, I went through a period of deep introspection. Why was I being so unlike my normal self? Why was I snapping at my spouse and children so readily? Why could I not control my irritable behavior making life less enjoyable for the people most important to me? How long would these symptoms last, and would they ever go away? And my deepest concern, would Kindra eventually pack her stuff and head out the door? These were my questions as I thought seriously about how to move forward. That's when I came up with an idea. I remembered our in-depth conversation by the walking trail just a few months earlier. We spent hours talking about the accident and my desire to teach again. So I invited Kindra to another important conversation in the great outdoors.

Setting a specific time and date for our discussion would not be a good idea since I never knew when the PCS symptoms would show up or how harsh they would be. That is why I decided an extemporaneous approach; a time when the symptoms were at a lower level would be best. I would invite Kindra to a stroll out by the lake so we could have another heart-to-heart conversation. We lived about 10 miles from an expansive lake complete with barbecue pits, boat ramps, and plenty of fishing. There were picnic tables scattered about with the peace and quiet needed for anyone desirous of some respite. It would be the perfect environment for broaching an extremely difficult but necessary conversation.

When the time was right, Kindra happily accepted my invitation, and we headed to the lake that very day. As expected, a calming breeze was blowing through the area, rustling some nearby trees and moving fallen leaves across the mostly empty parking area. I didn't waste any time at all letting Kindra know of my intentions. I wanted to talk about the accident, my behaviors since that time, and how they made her feel. I had her complete attention as I shared what I believed would be the perfect opening to a meaningful conversation: "Please tell me why you were crying the other night." She started in straight away as we moved across the dam and then along the lakeshore. It was a long path perfect for a lengthy and meaningful conversation.

The evening turned out better than I could have imagined, with respectful dialogue that set a new course for our relationship moving forward. We even talked about boundaries and provided "escape" options if my irritability became too much for her. Most people become irritable now and again; it's part of being human. However, with the brain-injured person, repeated episodes of irritability can wreak havoc on significant relationships. That is why, at the proper time and place, a deep and respectful conversation is important. A long-distance walk next to a lakeshore may not be best for every relationship, but it worked for ours. Whatever works best in your relationship, also be open to the help of a professional counselor.

Our new boundaries were set and worked well in our relationship. That's not to say that everything was smooth from the outset, but we were committed to making things work over time. We determined that two basic facts existed. Namely, that irritability following a head injury is common and difficult to control. Also, that an ongoing and persistent irritability can make a life partner feel extremely vulnerable and uncomfortable in the relationship. That is why I determined that when my PCS symptoms were at their worst, Kindra would simply use the opportunity to get some alone time. That is to say, she would spend a few hours with a close friend, head to the gym, visit the local library, do some shopping, or take Akaira out for a long walk. The possibilities are endless for the creative person, and Kindra went to several places over many months as I continued to heal.

If you've found yourself in the throes of your symptoms, and your significant relationships have suffered as a result, take heart. While everyone's journey is unique, and the symptoms can be incredibly difficult to manage, there is always hope if one is willing. We have definitely struggled, especially when the PCS symptoms have been at the worst, but we've managed to draw closer to one another through it all. And after all this time, we still incorporate the use of our boundary system whenever it becomes necessary. The PCS symptoms are less frequent now, but when they return, we have a plan in place to help keep our relationship on a respectful level.

Our walk by the lake was another pivotal point in our relationship, helping to prepare us for some very challenging days. If your relationship is currently in survival mode because of the ongoing symptoms of PCS, you may need to have that all-important conversation as well. If you haven't already set boundaries and/or sought out the help of an excellent counselor, maybe this is your next best step. Although our boundary system wasn't perfect in the beginning, requiring some fairly lengthy conversations, it eventually evolved into something workable and actually helped to make our relationship stronger.

Part of improving your situation is recognizing your symptoms for what they are; they are the result of an unexpected head injury. They are not the real you, never have been and never will be. The real you, the core of who you are, is not defined by your accident or manifestation, thereof. You are the same person you've always been. This doesn't mean that you will be able to overcome your irritability by willing it away. If the process were that easy, there would be no need for the encouragement of a friend, loved one, or professional counselor. There would be no need for books like this one or support groups where others share similar stories. In fact, according to the NIH, over 69 million people incur head injuries around the world each year. It's considered a silent epidemic as science continues its effort to address the many resulting problems, such as PCS.

There is a bottom line to all of this. That is, the individual who has sustained a head injury has only one choice, to overcome. That is it. There is no alternative. Don't let the darkness (anxiety, depression, irritability, forgetfulness, and headaches) become your vanguard. Choose wisely and remember the time-honored adage about the pebble in the pond. Your life does have influence, a powerful effect on those around you. Choose to learn all you can about your condition, include an excellent team of professionals that can help you, and be patient in the process. All of this is important in your effort to maintain a strong circle of family and friends as you continue on your healing journey.

There are often people who enter your life that might as well be part of your *family*. Some of these individuals might even become part of your *inner circle* at some point. I have not known Patti Foster for long, but her story of survival and hope has been a true inspiration to me. Truth be told, she has inspired thousands of people with head injuries all over the world through her public speaking, books, interviews, and other work. Patti sustained a head injury that went far beyond anything I have experienced. I definitely do not diminish the life-altering struggles of people who've sustained a mild TBI; however, my personal injury pales in comparison to what Patti has endured. After being left for dead, she not only survived but is thriving, offering hope to countless people around the world. Patti briefly shared her journey:

> It was about 6:40 in the evening on that hot, summer's night—June 18, 2002. . . over 100 degrees! Four of us ladies were in a red Tahoe, on our way to meet the others . . . Envision this with me: Emily had completely stopped her Tahoe at the red light [and] all lanes of traffic were full. I was sitting in the seat behind the driver [and] had just taken off my seatbelt to turn and check on some flowers I had bought for all the ladies in the Bible study (This was our last meeting before taking a summer break). The small bouquets of flowers were in a basket behind my seat where that storage area is in most SUVs. Then, all of a sudden, with no warning, *BAM!* The impact happened.
>
> A tractor-trailer rig pulling a trailer full of cars was barreling down the highway at 70 mph (67 mph, to be exact). It slammed into the rear of our completely stopped Tahoe with no slowing down. That cruel collision brought the vivacious life of this former radio personality to an abrupt halt! The right side of my face and head were crushed; my right eye was hanging out of its fractured orifice onto the highway, in a rapidly growing pool of my own blood. Fractures and

multiple injuries were all over me, from the top of my head to the tips of my toes. I had lost well over 60% of my blood and more than 20% of my body's tissue.

Am EMS worker searched for my pulse [with] no pulse to be found. So the white sheet was pulled over my body, assuming I was dead. As EMS staff raced against time to save lives, one of the eyewitnesses heard a gurgling noise coming from beneath that white sheet.

The second air-flight helicopter was contacted. After it had landed at the crash scene, the Flight Medic and Flight Nurse were attempting to load me onto the emergency helicopter. Despite all their efforts, my brain and body shut down and fell into a long-lasting coma. The pilot flew my comatose body to the nearest acute, hospital trauma-center. And for six weeks my brain and body lay in a coma, as my family was told I would be a persistent vegetable *if* I lived. I've had to re-learn every, single basic function of living . . . the crash instantly turned me into a 34-year-old infant.

Although Patti still struggles with her injuries, she has surpassed the expectations of her entire medical team. She continues to speak around the world, sharing her story of survival and pointing to hope. Patti emphasizes that brain injuries are often referred to as "invisible" since changes are on the inside. That is, others can't see your debilitating pain, disorientation, depression, anxiety, and a host of other issues. As someone whose heart literally stopped after a horrific accident, her story represents faith because that was her foundation. Her story represents hope because hope carried her through another day. And her story represents love because love is what it's all about. She is an example to the throngs of survivors and points to a peaceful respite, just over the horizon. For Patti Foster, King David's psalm glistened as she crossed over from death unto life:

> The Lord is my shepherd, I lack for nothing.
> He makes me lie down in green pastures,
> he leads me beside quiet waters,
> he refreshes my soul.
> He guides me along right paths
> for his name's sake.
> Even though I walk
> through the darkest valley,
> I will fear no evil,
> for you are with me;
> your rod and your staff,
> they comfort me.
> You prepare a table before me
> in the presence of my enemies.
> You anoint my head with oil;
> my cup overflows.
> Surely your goodness and love will follow me
> all the days of my life,
> And I will dwell in the house of the LORD
> forever.
>
> (Psalm 23, NLT)

People with head injuries need others in their lives that will support them every step of the way. It's definitely not for the faint of heart but well worth the effort within healthy and loving relationships. In my healing journey, I needed the comfort and encouragement of my wife. I needed the occasional phone call from my mother, brothers, and friends. I needed the uplifting words from counselors and pastors. I needed what became a small community of caring people who spoke into my life words of support. And I also needed inspiration from people like Patti Foster to complete the circle.

Meanwhile, our journey is ongoing. The clouds continue their ominous presence, sometimes overshadowing our hope for normalcy and peace. But it's not the gathering of those dark clouds with their message of discontent; it's the peering of sunlight breaking through the clouds, just above the mountaintops. We know it's there because we can see it. We can feel it. We are reaching out for hope because hope *doesn't disappoint*. The doom and despair that are sometimes associated with PCS cannot win. Victory belongs to the one who overcomes, not letting anguish rule the soul. Reach out to those friends and family members who love and care for you. No matter the size of your caring community, those individuals who truly love you embrace those relationships as part of your holistic approach to healing.

6

Post-Concussion Syndrome and Finances

I once heard a medical practitioner refer to brain injury as the "ultimate disrupter." Just about every facet of life within the family context can be affected after a brain injury, and depending on the severity and location of the specific injury, disruptions can range from minor to significant. As of late, I'm not sure where I fall on the PCS symptom scale, but I do experience symptoms that are overwhelming at times. My family and I had just moved to a different part of the country and were excited about new possibilities when a horrible traffic accident changed just about everything, including our finances. One of the biggest hurdles that families face following an unexpected brain injury is the stability of finances. Often, the injured family member is a major contributor to household finances, creating a substantial burden when they can no longer work full-time.

Household budgets can be disrupted in any number of ways, including inability to work following an accident. And when the accident involves a head injury of some sort, returning to work becomes a real challenge. In fact, workers who develop PCS following a head injury are sometimes only able to return part-time or not at all. Even if the head-injured family member wasn't working before

10.4324/9781003216056-6

the accident, the financial toll can be devastating. When my car was broadsided, I was not thinking about our family budget. I was headed to my son's school, and he was ready to go home. The accident only took a few seconds, but it created a ripple effect that touched every part of our lives and those immediately around us. Just a few seconds in time and we were forced to rethink our entire family structure, including how we would address our financial needs moving forward.

When we strolled the streets of Eden, I was working close to 50 hours per week and dedicated to hard work each and every day. As a new high school vice principal, I was being paid to attend trainings, write a career handbook, help with employment policies, and do any other tasks as assigned by my supervisor. I was also teaching an online graduate research course as my second job. I was gainfully employed, as many people are when their lives are suddenly turned upside down after a tragic accident. I never imagined that life could change as quickly as it did. My mild TBI and subsequent PCS had a direct effect on our family roles, schedules, communication, work responsibilities, and so much more.

Having a good work ethic was instilled into me when I was very young. My parents taught me the importance of working hard through the example they set in everyday life. My dad worked hard at the local plywood mill, which employed over 600 people at one location. The superintendent at the plant recognized my dad's hard work and promoted him several times, eventually landing him the second-highest role of assistant superintendent. My dad was responsible for giving me my first "real" job that came complete with good wages and benefits to eventually take care of my own family. His only request was that

I show up to the jobsite every day, work hard, and treat other employees with respect.

Working in a plywood mill was not easy. Inside the plant were six giant dryers, each the size of a small house. The dryers were used to remove moisture from countless sheets of wood veneer during each of the three shifts. Although the dryers only represented a small percentage of machinery in the building, they contributed to the stifling heat during the summertime. When the outside temperature was unbearably hot, the veneer dryers became a catalyst in raising the inside temperature even higher. Our supervisors did not care much about the uncomfortable weather; they expected high levels of production, stifling heat or not. Along with the example set by my parents, the mill provided an excellent opportunity to learn the value of hard work as an ongoing commitment to taking care of my family.

Unfortunately, before I ever learned the significance of being an adult and staying committed to a job, my mother found herself alone to raise five sons without the help of a life partner. Raising children is not easy for two people, let alone one. I was 11 years old when everything went down, and it rocked my world. It rocked everyone in our family, but especially Mom. When one person in a family unit is no longer around, it has a dramatic effect on the dynamic of that family, especially if the individual now absent happens to be a parent. Add that to the shift in roles and responsibilities, and the emotional toll for everyone was significant.

Mom eventually came to grips with her situation and sat down to make plans. The facts were clear; she had five children and a long list of monthly obligations. The mortgage payment alone would overwhelm anyone, but she determined to make things work. Her job at the hospital would not be enough, so she took on a second job at a local convenience store. She also adjusted her monthly budget where she could and reluctantly accepted help to fill in the gaps. I remember that our roles changed almost immediately. My eldest brother, Buzz, for example, was no longer simply the firstborn of five sons. He was now partly responsible for making sure his younger brothers were safe and well cared for while Mom put in some very long hours at work.

My brothers and I admired Mom's tenacity for gearing into survival mode. I still do not know exactly how she pulled it off, but she did. Even after several years have passed, I'm in awe of her raw strength and aspire to emulate her in my own life. Like my mother, my world has been rocked and thrown into disarray, but I am following her incredible example on how to navigate the most troubling of waters. President John F. Kennedy's father, Joseph P. Kennedy, is well known for this statement: "When life gets tough, the tough get going." And certainly, my mother is one of the toughest people I know. I determined a long time ago to follow her lead ensuring the best possible outcome after my car accident and the PCS that followed.

Having an exemplar in your life means far more than being inspired by a favorite sports team or motivational speaker. I had a front-row seat as my mom grappled with challenges, not knowing if she would succeed from one day to the next. It was her abiding faith that failure was not an option moving her to place one foot in front of the other, even through the growing list of uncertainties. Through it all, she crossed the finish line and is now realizing the fruits of her hard labor. Her children are raised with children of their own. Her mortgage is completely paid off, and she has food on the table. She has even traveled around the world and accomplished dreams she never thought possible.

The loss of a stable household income, whether through death, divorce, head injury, or some other unexpected event, can bring a great deal of distress into a family. The sooner finances are put in order, the better. In their review of the effects of job loss and unemployment on families, McKee-Ryan and Maitoza (2014) conclude the following:

- Unemployment affects the unemployed worker, his or her partner or spouse, and other household members in addition to disrupting the family system.
- Unemployment may trigger a cascade of additional stressors to the family system that need to be addressed simultaneously. Among these stressors is the possibility of changed family roles and family dynamics.
- Family members and spouses need to recognize that the experience of unemployment is stressful for the job seeker and that their interaction with him or her can help or hinder the process of becoming reemployed. In particular, family members can bolster the self-confidence of the job seeker, provide practical advice and support for job seeking, and help the job seeker stay actively involved in the job-search process. Although families may experience financial distress, reminding the job seeker of the financial shortfall and the need for reemployment can inhibit rather than encourage reemployment.
- Unemployed workers need to remain emotionally involved with their family members. Although being unemployed typically means that the unemployed worker will be at home and physically present more often, that does not automatically translate into being emotionally present for family members.

- Children in the home may need reassurance from parents relating to the following:

  o The fact that the child was not responsible for the job loss

  o Making the child feel secure and reminding the child that the world remains a safe place, and

  o Modeling work behavior and positive attitudes toward work so that the child maintains positive expectations about future employment opportunities and continues to see the importance of investing efforts into educational pursuits.

  (Job Loss, Unemployment, and Families, 2018, p. 95)

Without question, a brain injury is the "ultimate disrupter." Even for people suffering from mild TBI, the financial challenges can be daunting. My wife and I were excited about my new position at the high school. Accepting the job meant that our family income would increase, providing a better outlook for our family. The accident not only returned us to a place substantially below our previous income level, it added unexpected challenges with the PCS symptoms and increased medical bills. Because sustainable income is such an important part of family life, affecting even the basic needs of survival, sustainability should be addressed as soon as possible. A lack of financial peace within the home complicates the head-injured family member's road to recovery and the overall health of the family unit. In her research, Brand (2015) discusses the implications of job loss, which can include an array of challenges such as a "[h]igher level of depressive symptoms and poor health" (p. 13).

If you or someone in your family has sustained a serious head injury, and your financial budget has been affected, it's time to make some changes. The most important consideration is an accounting of your daily, weekly, and monthly obligations. You'll need to know your exact bottom line. What is the minimum amount of money you will need each month to survive? Has your monthly income changed since your accident? Following my accident, I went from working approximately 50 hours per week down to 17 hours per week. Aside from the injuries, the immediate result of my accident was the loss of 60% of our total household income.

Maybe the repercussions from your accident have been more complicated than mine. Some accident victims are the sole providers in their respective homes and have, in essence, lost 100% of their income. The spectrum is as wide as the number of people sustaining head injuries around the world each year. It's a serious problem needing serious consideration. In order to know precisely how to address the issue, you'll need to take account of your specific circumstance, no matter how troublesome it might be. The first step is a simple as an itemized budget. This type of budget will cover the important categories and will provide an accurate snapshot moving forward. While it's true that most people already have a working budget in place before an accident, it's imperative that the budget be readdressed if the income has been impacted.

If you have access to the Internet or local library, there are resources to help you in setting up a new itemized budget. And of course, there are apps around the world that can add a high level of efficiency to the process. Many apps go beyond the basics of debt-to-income accounting. For example, in the UK, Money Dashboard is considered one of the top apps for budgeting purposes. Money Dashboard was voted Best Personal Finance App and helps users connect bank accounts, categorize spending, create an offline account, set budgets, set up payday cycles, transfer money, predict balances, set goals, and more. Money Dashboard and other UK apps, such as Yolt and Emma, are free to users. In the US, Mint is a viable option that stands out as user-friendly and free to use. Other apps, such as simplifi and PocketGuard, are also free and excellent tools for closely monitoring your budget.

After taking a close look at your budget, consider making an appointment with a financial planner. Financial planners typically specialize in defined areas, but you'll need one that will provide a plan that helps you get back on your feet. Unfortunately, many head-injured patients find themselves in a situation where they can't even afford the cost of a financial planner. If this is true for you and your family, many countries provide free or low-cost assistance to help make reasonable, goal-oriented plans for success. One example of an organization in the UK offering free debt advice is Consumer Credit Counseling Services. Similarly, in the US, credit counseling agencies are available that provide services for free or at a very low cost. If you live outside the UK and the US, perform diligent research to learn what might be available in your area. Even if you are adept in financial management, it won't hurt to run ideas by another professional. Maybe they can offer suggestions that you had not considered.

It is important that you communicate with someone in the financial community to help set your mind at ease, even if the professional is someone close to you, such as a relative or family friend. Unless you were financially viable before the accident, including several months of emergency funds on reserve, you will need some outside advice on the best way to move forward. Sometimes the objective opinion of someone who works in the financial industry can be incredibly helpful, both for budgeting purposes and to give you a sense of hope moving forward. You are in a new and very challenging life situation that will require your full attention and dedication. But the old saying is true: "This too shall pass," and it will. There are count-less people around the world, including my own mother, who've faced incredible odds and came out stronger on the other end. You can too.

Your financial planner will likely ask you to consider downsizing. Downsizing is not easy, especially if you've been working hard at upsizing in recent years. Every dollar that can be saved by lowering expenses should be saved. And depending on your personal situation, more difficult decisions, such as moving to a less expensive home, might need to happen. These are not easy decisions, but remem-ber, this is where the *rubber meets the road* on your path back to normalcy. Your financial planner will likely sug-gest additional consideration, such as comparison shop-ping for food, taking another look at your phone service, carpooling if possible, paying in cash, and eating out less often or not at all. The creative person can find unique ways to accommodate a budget after a major hit to the bottom line.

In addition to cutting monthly expenditures, consider looking at additional income possibilities. If your country or local municipality offers some sort of unemployment assistance program, see if you qualify for that assistance. For some people, this will require they set aside their hon-orable practice of self-sufficiency. Everyone needs help at some point in life. If you have been the major provider for yourself and your family, do not feel ashamed to ask someone else for help as you work toward getting back on your feet, especially after an unexpected accident of some sort; it might be your turn to reach out for help. Be willing to allow others to help you for a change. Because of your injuries, if you are unable to increase your workload at the present time, consider all your possible options, including disability income, if that type of assistance is available in your area.

If you have not already applied for or received disability assistance from your country or municipality, it might be worth your time to research this possibility. Some countries offer programs meant to help people with unemployment or disability needs. Countries like Estonia, France, Germany, Ireland, Italy, Japan, Russia, South Africa, and the Nordic countries have programs in place that are considered some of the best in the world. Of course, the UK and the US have special programs as well to assist with unemployment and/or disability needs. In the UK, PIP (Personal Independence Payment) helps with costs associated with long-term disability. Other programs, such as Disability Premiums, Disabled Persons and Work, and Specialist Employability Support, help fill in the gaps for other unemployment and disability-related needs. In the US, visit usa.gov, then key in "find government and local disability programs and services." Many other counties offer similar benefits to help their citizens with unemployment and disability needs.

In my own journey with mild TBI, my goal has always been to return to full-time employment when and if I could. All the way back to my experience in the plywood mill, even when the temperatures were unbearably hot, I loved being gainfully employed and participating as part of a productive team environment. There is something special about working toward a common goal. Equally fulfilling is being a provider of the financial needs of your home. Whether one is working as a janitor at the local high school or chief executive officer of a major corporation, work brings about a sense of accomplishment—accomplishment that can bless an entire family. Unfortunately, like many people dealing with PCS, I haven't been able to return to work full-time. This reality created an added burden, not just for my own emotional well-being but for the health of our household budget as well. We had to make serious changes that required rethinking every aspect of our financial lives.

Following my brain injury, we learned early on that we'd need to make some changes if we were going to be successful. As a first step in our journey, we met with a financial adviser for ideas on how we might move forward. She was wonderful and offered useful ideas on how to stay afloat. We followed her advice closely since failure was not an option no matter what obstacles we had to face. We agreed with our counselor that new employment for Kindra with improved pay and benefits should be considered. And since we had already determined to head for the southern United States, we looked for positions in the central and northern parts of Texas. In our case, we were fortunate that Kindra worked in the high-demand area of healthcare, so she was offered a new position in a relatively short period of time.

Moving to a different location with a lower cost of living (in most communities) and no state income tax was a good move for us. We found a community that offered highly rated schools and a beautiful environment in which to live and explore. We also followed the steps laid out in this chapter, such as assessing our budget in order to prioritize our expenses. Like many households, we also carried debt, which added to our anxiety levels after the accident. Our financial counselor reassured us that a solid plan would reduce our stress levels and actually provide direction moving forward. In fact, some of our creditors agreed to accept smaller monthly payments until we could restabilize our household income. The goal is to begin with baby steps until you can stabilize every area of your family budget. This will take time and concerted effort for you and/or your family, but it can be done.

According to a survey conducted by the American Psychological Association (APA), money is the top cause of stress for families. In fact, according to Dr. Linda Gallo (2015), "Stress can negatively affect health and even contribute to chronic health problems such as diabetes and heart disease" (para. 1). Given that money, or more precisely, the lack thereof, can play such a significant role in the psychological and physical health of the individual, it's imperative that one's "house" be placed in order following TBI. Along with the suggestions presented in this chapter, seeking out the help of a professional adviser/counselor can go a long way toward your goal of stability in your household budget.

Whether your objective is to increase your working hours from none to part-time or part-time to full-time, make it your ambition to bring peace to your household budget in the interim. Do whatever needs to be done to bring stability to your home. Head injuries complicate a great many areas of family life. The entire family dynamic changes after a loved one sustains a serious head injury. Individual family roles, responsibilities, and communication are all affected. Do your best to improve your household income and debt situation so that you can realize more peace within a stable and peaceful home environment.

7

Post-Traumatic Stress Disorder

As a new arrival at Fort Campbell, it's a real challenge to feel *at home* with so much going on overseas. Terrorism had struck the homeland, and new military recruits were signing up every day. Also feeling compelled to join the cause was my daughter, Rachael, who had just finished her Army basic and advanced infantry training. Located on the Tennessee-Kentucky state line in the United States, Fort Campbell would be her first duty assignment and where she'd be part of something bigger than herself. Home to the 101st Airborne Division and 160th Special Operations Aviation Regiment, the base is considered a stalwart for the United States military housing over 200,000 active-duty personnel, family, and support.

New arrivals to Fort Campbell were told to report to the screening station at the Kalsu Replacement Company. The soldiers were processed and sent immediately to their assigned posts. The entire operation took about 14 days, including the orientation, team briefs, medical, dental, and haircuts. Rachael had given herself a clear objective; keep a low profile, meet every expectation, and prepare to impress. Unfortunately, things didn't quite work out the way she'd hope. She forgot to bring along her medical forms and found herself being loudly shouted down by an officer in front of an entire room of soldiers. Her goal of

10.4324/9781003216056-7

proving her metal over the first few days had seemingly been dismantled in one setting. It was an embarrassing moment that left her reeling and wondering if she'd even succeed.

That's when she saw him. It was the very same soldier she noticed previously standing near a picnic table between the male and female barracks. Only this time, there would be no admiring from a distance. This guy was on a mission and headed straight toward her. "Let me give you a ride to your barracks to grab up your papers, and we'll get you right back here." Rachael was taken aback but decided to accept the invitation, given the unexpected attention she'd received just moments earlier. But little did she know, the brief ride with this unidentified soldier would be the foundation to something much more.

The idea of falling in love is a strange and mysterious thing. It's a phenomenon hard to describe save for a handful of well-seasoned poets. What about a timeline for falling in love? The lilies of Britain take a hundred days to blossom. Is it the same for true love? Maybe the troubadours of France had it right when they professed just a glimpse into another's eyes might kindle love at first sight. Whatever the case, Rachael was very curious about this soldier and wanted to see him again. Her feelings were hard to explain, but they were real. Call it an attraction or simple infatuation; this person had commanded her thoughts for the next several days.

The extended Fourth of July weekend finally arrived, and nearly everyone had left the base leaving it quiet and unsettled. With spare time on her hands, Rachael decided to head outdoors to take in some sunshine. She really had no master plan that afternoon, but taking a walk would be a great place to start. As a fairly new arrival to the base, she hadn't yet had an opportunity to check out the natural beauty she had heard so much about. Fort Campbell had plenty to offer by way of plant life with native grasslands, agriculture fields, and forests. The woodland areas alone included over 48,000 acres. Of course, she wouldn't be able to see much in one day, but a brief look around would do her some good.

As Rachael was making her way past the common area between the male and female barracks, she spotted the same soldier who sparked her interest. She hesitated for a moment remembering the shellacking she took in front of this person back at the replacement company. Always the introspective thinker, she made the immediate decision that it was best to quickly and quietly fades into the tree line. She almost made it, too, when she heard the man's voice calling: "Don't leave!" The soldier ran up to her and coaxed her back to the picnic area. Their conversation was not the usual introductory pleasantries and small talk. It seemed they had everything in common. And Rachael's new interest, Casey Watters, ended the conversation that evening by stating, "Well, Red, I guess we're hanging out this weekend!"

Over the Fourth of July weekend, they spent every available moment together, but it all started with an official date. Driving an old pickup truck, complete with lifted frame and roll cage, Casey showed up at Rachael's barrack's door and knocked. Rachael had been mulling how much she and this man had in common but never imagined this self-proclaimed strongman would show up carrying a bouquet of flowers. It was clear that he had fallen for her and had one objective on this evening, to impress. He walked her to his truck and opened the passenger door. His first act of kindness set the stage for an evening that was surprisingly pleasant. That is, until a giant misstep landed Rachael into a hospital emergency room later that night.

Casey wanted to impress Rachael, and flowers didn't seem quite enough. She was intelligent, and her quick wit made him feel he was outgunned in casual conversation. And there was something about the way she carried herself that left him flummoxed and losing his train of thought. So as they were driving out of the restaurant parking lot, Casey decided to put the pedal to the mettle. That's right—he pushed the gas pedal to the floor to demonstrate his Andretti-like skills with tires screeching and smoke billowing. It was a made-for-television scene that went nearly perfect until a piece of his truck clipped the concrete base of a nearby light post. What started out as a perfect first date, complete with roses and laughter, ended with Rachael needing immediate treatment at a nearby hospital emergency room.

Not even a trip to the emergency room could dissuade Rachael from continuing to spend time with her new interest. They spent every available moment together when they weren't attending training or some other active duty requirement. It was a whirlwind courtship in full force when the mobilization alert came. It's not as though they weren't thinking about the possibility in the back of their minds, after all; it's something soldiers think about often. But when they did receive their orders, it was like a ton of bricks landed squarely on their hopes of spending more time together. Rachael's orders read that she was being deployed to Camp Anaconda, now referred to as Joint Base Balad, Joint Operations Base, in Balad, Iraq. Casey, on the other hand, was being assigned to the infamous 187th Infantry Regiment (Rakkasans), also in Iraq. They might as well have been assigned an ocean apart because they likely wouldn't see one another for a very long time.

Everything was so very secretive; it was part of the war-time motif. The less said, the less likely a soldier would get into trouble. Soldiers were highly trained and knew a level of secrecy was baked into the process. However, once things kicked into high gear, it was like a locomotive barreling down the tracks, intent on its destination. "You just did what you had to do" is how Rachael described the process. Each soldier was given a list and needed to check each box prior to deployment. There were medical and legal requirements and everything in between. It all had to get done. It was an arduous process, but one requirement caused Rachael to think deeply about her journey ahead; she had to write down her own will. The entire process took place within hours, and before she knew it, she was on a bus headed for Virginia to catch her flight out.

When soldiers are sent overseas, they don full uniforms and keep weapons at their sides. As a female soldier, Rachael was required to have her long red hair placed in a bun and tucked under her Kevlar. These requirements are ongoing, even as they take civilian flights to their final destinations. Rachael noted a comment she heard the pilot make on her commercial flight just before takeoff: "Ladies and gentlemen, please ensure your weapons are stored by your feet with the muzzles pointed toward the cockpit." The announcement was a nice distraction, but Rachael couldn't stop thinking about Casey. She studied a few pictures on her cell phone but was already feeling emptiness in the pit of her stomach. It was a deep kind of longing that made her wonder about the future and what it would hold, especially given they were both being assigned to a battle zone.

Rachael's journey from an airport in Virginia included several layover flights partly due to "aircraft technical malfunctions," but she finally arrived at Camp Wolf in Kuwait. Her stay at the base lasted a few short days before she was flown out via C-130 military aircraft to her destination in Mosul, Iraq. However, before even landing at Camp Wolf, she jotted her contact information on a piece of paper in hopes she would come across a soldier in the terminal wearing a Screaming Eagle's insignia. If a soldier were wearing that specific insignia, it would mean he was part of the same elite group as Casey in the 187th Infantry Regiment.

Rachael spotted a soldier with the insignia and approached him. "Please don't think I'm crazy. I'm trying to find someone." She pulled the paper from her pocket and handed it to him. "I know it's a lot to ask, but if you run across a PFC Casey Watters at the 187th, would you give this to him? I'd be forever grateful." Rachael knew chances were slim given the size of Casey's division, but she was desperate. The soldier said he'd try, but that wasn't enough for Rachael. She made her way to the concession area, ordered a light lunch, and quickly jotted a few more notes. Finding a Screaming Eagle in the terminal wouldn't be easy, but she was able to distribute one more message with her contact information.

Rachael never heard back from Casey and was eventually flown to her final destination at the Joint Operations Base in Balad, Iraq. As a new arrival, she was pleasantly surprised to learn that Anaconda, as it was commonly called, was one of the best military base facilities in Iraq and had access to swimming pools, restaurants, snack bars, and even dancing lessons. But her short-lived excitement for what was definitely *le meilleur* of the US military's bases turned sour as she quickly learned the dangers of serving in a war zone. She was just settling in and feeling optimistic about her accommodations when she walked to the DFAC ("dee-fac"), or local dining facility, for some lunch.

The chow line heading into the facility was ridiculous. The line of soldiers was so long it wrapped around the block and joined up with a second extended line. Rachael thought to herself, "This is my life now for the next few months, so I've got to be patient and adapt." However, patience wouldn't be the first word that comes to mind after what happened next. As she was just turning the corner in front of a building, mortars came raining down. With mortars, there's usually no warning sound as they can cover the distance between a launch site and the target faster than the human ear can perceive. For Rachael and the other soldiers in the line, it would have been a complete surprise. This was her first exposure to live fire and likely the first for most of the other soldiers in the line.

After the first mortar hit, Rachael noticed the troops staying put and staring at one another. Her heart started beating faster as she wondered if this was a normal part of the daily routine? "We get in line, wait for chow, and get bombed? That's how life works at Anaconda? Are we're just supposed to hope that each day is not our last?" Rachael tried to make sense of what was happening but couldn't. After another three or four explosions, a group of infantry personnel ran through the area shouting loudly, "What the hell is wrong with you people? TAKE COVER!" Just then, everyone in the line ran in different directions looking for a safe shelter of some kind. Anaconda was an old Iraqi air base and had multiple buildings scattered about that were formed in concrete. Rachael spotted one of these structures directly across the street and quickly ran in that direction. Just as she turned behind one of the walls, she felt the shockwaves of a concussive blast radiate through her body.

Rachael stated, "[I]t's heat and pressure, like your organs are slamming into half of your body as the energy moves through you, it's indescribably intense." She continued in what she called an Anaconda baptism by fire: "I'll never forget coming out of the shelter. It was my first experience being that close to enemy fire and I was in a daze. For some reason [I was thinking] that I needed to get back out there before the line gets crazy long again. Once I reentered the glaring sunlight, I surveyed the damage. I noticed a giant black crater on the corner in front of the chow hall, exactly where I was standing." Rachael felt blessed to be alive but didn't yet realize this event would be the first of several, laying the foundation for her developing nightmare of post-traumatic stress disorder (PTSD).

In another experience at Anaconda, Rachael talked about perimeter guard duty, something she had done a few times. Guarding the outer portion of the base provided the first line of defense, alerting others of potential threats. Guards were stationed in nests while on the lookout for enemy combatants.

> There was one time I was up there when a cart pulled by a donkey slowly [made] its way near our area. As I sat there . . . I heard a vehicle approaching. It was maybe two seconds later that I felt the air being displaced next to my head, and then heard the crack of the shot. After taking cover, my battle buddy and I immediately radioed in the attack and prepared to return fire . . . Our Quick Response Team (QRT) confirmed they were on the way. We took on heavy fire until the man with the donkey and the diversionary truck made their escape. Later, while examining the scene, I noticed a bullet in the back of my tower area that had hit about two inches above where my head had been.

Soldiers who served in battle zones often develop PTSD from their life-threatening experiences. The symptoms for these soldiers often include reoccurring intrusive reminders of the traumatic event and extreme avoidance of anything that might bring back memories of that event. Also, the individual might experience negative changes in thoughts and mood, as well as guardedness and emotional reactions to certain situations. When your daily life includes the potential for danger, such as serving in a war zone or being physically abused by someone who's supposed to care, there is the possibility of developing PTSD. However, for Rachael, there was one particular encounter that rocked her emotions more than any other.

Rachael has mostly blocked from her memory much of what happened on that day, but she remembers the basic construct:

> We were in [a particular] province delivering supplies, which was part of my duty while serving over there. I was keeping my head on a swivel watching for any potential threats or danger. Then I noticed a small child, who had come into my periphery, then turned to take a closer look. I remember thinking the child was adorable, but I quickly refocused since we were in a dangerous sector. Staying on high alert and being vigilant was critical if you wanted to come home alive. Right after I had those thoughts, all hell broke loose. It turned out the child was a plant and was fitted with some type of explosive device. It was a suicide-bombing situation that we'd heard so much about. It was heartbreaking that the child, along with a group of people standing nearby, were killed.

Rachael doesn't recall more detail about that day, but she does remember the emotional aspect of it all. That is often the case with PTSD; details about the trauma somehow get blocked from memory while the basic framework of the event might still be intact. That's the way it is with post-traumatic stress. Rachael remembers feeling a sense of terror after the bomb went off and feeling like she would probably die. There's also a deep and inner concern for your friends and if they'll survive the ordeal. She stated,

> You don't think, you simply do. Then afterwards shaking like you are freezing cold, but not being cold. Of being so relieved it's over, but looking around seeing the damage, and feeling like you failed. You're exhausted. Being so tired you want to give up, but not doing so because you want your friends to be OK. Wanting to sleep, but not being able to. To this day I still can't sleep, and the tiredness has never left.

Rachael's overseas obligation at Anaconda lasted one year. In all that time, she never heard from Casey and often wondered how he was doing. Several stressful life-threatening encounters of her own made her wonder if Casey was even alive since he would have experienced even closer encounters with the enemy. These are the kinds of thoughts one has when there's simply no credible information to assuage such concerns. But now that she was headed back to the United States, she could do some investigative work while life wasn't so hectic. After all that time, she still got butterflies in her stomach when thinking about him but had no indication that he was still interested in her.

Casey joined the military in response to the terrorist attacks against the United States on September 11, 2001. Like Rachael, he understood that the Iraqis were wonderful people with their own families, friends, and aspirations for the future. However, like many regions of the world, there were also factions bent on ideological lawlessness. But Casey's was a call to duty, an inner desire to join a cause in protecting the viability of law-abiding citizens. It's from that vantage that he felt a strong pull to be part of something bigger than himself. Freedom has never come easy, and Casey was willing to put his own life in harm's way to help ensure that future generations could live lives of stability and peace.

After completing his tour of duty in Iraq, Casey headed to the United States with one thing on his mind—the redhead. That was his personal moniker for Rachael, and she didn't take it as disrespect. The two eventually found one another again and got married within a relatively short period of time. They soon had a daughter and named her Cara, which was a combination of their two first names. Although both Casey and Rachael were having very real-life struggles with post-traumatic stress, Casey headed out for his second tour of duty. As a dedicated soldier, a special calling handed down from his father, Casey felt a need to help complete the mission.

Now that Casey was serving overseas again, Rachael decided to travel with young Cara to Alaska to stay with her mother for a while. This would help give her the kind of peace she needed while missing her husband and still struggling with the symptoms of PTSD. As well, Casey's mom decided to join them in Alaska, which provided even more support during some very trying times. However, Rachael recalls the exact time and date when her world was turned upside down in the middle of a timed period of respite. It was early in the morning on January 28, 2006, when she got the call. Casey was on the phone following an ambush his unit experienced while on patrol in Iraq:

> I was still laying there with this sense of dread when my cell rang around 2:00 a.m. It was my husband. He sounded amped up with what I now know was an adrenaline rush. Their convoy hit an improvised explosive device (IED), killing his best friend and roommate, SSG David Herrera, instantly. Casey had also been injured in the explosion, his body slammed into the roof of his Humvee with the left side of his neck absorbing most of the trauma. I found out later that he was actually a hero that day; most of the team ran out with him towards the lead vehicle SSG Herrera was in, leaving everyone exposed when the ambush started. Almost immediately one of his soldiers was shot in the head, but fortunately, he survived. Chaos and confusion abounded but Casey's cooler head prevailed. He immediately jumped on the radio, calling in and directing air support.

After Casey returned home to his family, he learned that his exposure to depleted uranium was the cause of a very rare cancer that would eventually take his life. The months that he had left with Rachael and Cara proved extremely challenging, dealing with not just the excruciating effects of cancer but also the PTSD. Rachael laid her husband to rest on June 17, 2009, when their daughter was just four years old. As one might imagine, she had a very difficult time readjusting to her life without the man whom she had fallen in love with from almost the first day. Even to this day, Rachael misses Casey and still struggles with the ongoing symptoms of PTSD, a disorder that probably began with a blast not far from a lunch line at Anaconda.

PTSD is a mental health condition that is most often associated with soldiers who've experienced or witnessed life-threatening events while serving in combat zones. However, PTSD can affect anyone who has been exposed to a traumatic event, whether it is through combat, vehicle accident, physical abuse, or some other life-threatening situation. According to the National Institute of Mental Health (NIMH), "It is natural to feel afraid during and after a traumatic situation. Fear triggers many split-second changes in the body to help defend against danger or to avoid it." Each person responds differently in their initial reaction to trauma, and some experience ongoing struggles that might eventually be diagnosed as PTSD. In determining if PTSD is present, a person must have all of the following for a period of at least one month (NIMH):

- At least one reexperiencing symptom
- At least one avoidance symptom
- At least two arousal and reactivity symptoms
- At least two cognition and mood symptoms.

The reexperiencing symptoms include the following:

- Flashbacks—reliving the trauma over and over, including physical symptoms like racing heart or sweating
- Bad dreams
- Frightening thoughts

The reoccurring symptoms of PTSD can be very disruptive to a person's everyday routines and can be triggered by thoughts or feelings. Individuals can also experience avoidance symptoms, which include staying away from places, events, or objects that are reminders of a traumatic event (NIMH).

According to the UK-based organization Mind, a person with PTSD might experience heightened alertness (hypervigilance) or "feeling on edge" as panic works its way in. They might also be angered, irritable, or aggressive and be jumpy or easily startled. Often, there's also a sense that no one else can truly understand the experience, except maybe others who've gone through the same type of life-threatening event. "This could be because when we feel stressed emotionally, our bodies release hormones called *cortisol* and *adrenaline*. This is the body's automatic way of preparing to respond to a threat, sometimes called the 'fight, flight or freeze' response" (Mind.org). Post-traumatic stress produces these hormones even when real danger is no longer present.

The number of people who suffer worldwide from war-related PTSD and major depression could be as high as 354 million (Hoppen & Morina, 2019). This number does not include those who develop the disorder through other life-threatening events, such as car accidents or physical abuse. Although a great deal has been learned about PTSD, the experience itself can feel far more than a clinical definition might ascribe. The dark experience can cause the individual to feel isolated, as though no one else could even minutely relate. Fear, uncertainty, and darkness set in like concrete, leaving the victim feeling trapped and abandoned. Earlier, I described the experience of visiting a cave system in the Pacific Northwest of the United States. After the tour guide extinguishes the light for just a moment, the darkness becomes so palpable and overwhelming it envelops your entire being, down to the lower reaches of your soul. The darkness is so tangible you can almost feel it on your skin.

While I worked in the plywood mill during my early career, I also volunteered as an emergency medical technician (EMT) for a local rescue organization. Rogue Ambulance Service no longer exists but was a notable rescue service in the area and covered 900 square miles within a southern Oregon territory of the United States. During my time with the organization, I responded to vehicle accidents, shooting victims, drowning, cardiac arrests, industrial accidents, fall victims, fires, assaults, and a host of other traumatic situations. I don't recall that I ever experienced any of the PTSD symptoms while working as an EMT. There was no agitation, irritability, insomnia, anxiety, depression, fear, or nightmares. I enjoyed helping others in need and felt confident in my ability to do so. However, after I was broadsided in an intersection several years later and sustained a head injury as a result, I experienced several of the symptoms over an extended period of time.

Although not previously referred to as such, PTSD goes back in the eons of time and has brushed against the famous, commoners, and even some found in literature around the world. In fact, according to the National Center for PTSD (in the US), Shakespeare's Henry IV appears to meet many, if not all, of the diagnostic criteria for PTSD (para. 1). However, it wasn't until the latter part of the 20th century that psychiatric organizations began to recognize the PTSD concept as an "etiological agent" existing outside the individual, as in a traumatic event. Previously, the condition was thought to be a traumatic neurosis, or inherent individual weakness. The evolution of understanding has provided a more appropriate diagnosis and led to a specific classification scheme helping to provide improved treatment for people suffering after a traumatic event.

After my car accident, I learned firsthand the stress that sometimes follows a traumatic event. It was powerful and not something I could fight with my own determination or raw grit. In my case, it only took one brief traumatic event to bring this beast (my definition) into my life. I can't even imagine the grip PTSD has over someone returning from the battlefield. Soldiers not only experience traumatic events, but they operate in harm's way, day in and day out. Whatever the cause of the PTSD, symptoms most often include vivid flashbacks, intrusive thoughts or images, nightmares, intense distress, and physical sensations (pain, sweating, nausea, trembling), which can take the sufferer to some dark places. But with the help of improved treatment strategies and people who really do care, there can be light at the end of a very long tunnel.

If you or someone in your family is suffering from PTSD, it's important to talk about what situations or specific conversations might trigger flashbacks or difficult feelings (Mind.org.uk). In some cases, it might be as simple as a loud noise, an argument, or a particular place that causes flashbacks or distressed feelings. The Mind approach to dealing with these types of situations is a proactive one. Families should plan ahead or even write down a crisis plan to help navigate the symptoms. In addition to the valuable resources provided by organizations like Mind, if you haven't already done so, consider including a counselor who is trained in PTSD and other issues that sometimes accompany such as anxiety and depression. Through cognitive behavioral therapy and other research-based approaches, there is hope for people struggling with PTSD.

Meanwhile, research and technology march ahead, providing even more hope for people suffering from PTSD and TBI. While the industrial revolution and engineering were the cornerstones of advancement a hundred years ago, the current century has seen self-driving cars, autonomous flying vehicles, and smartphones, among countless other innovations. In the grand perspective of time, so much has happened in relatively short order. In fact, while growing up, I remember my own mother and other people living in our neighborhood still drying laundry on clotheslines out in the open air. It's just one example of how technology has improved in the last few years, from the convenience of appliances to saving countless lives through medical breakthroughs in the scientific and research world.

Even the term *PTSD* didn't come into its own until 1980, when the term first appeared in the third edition of the *Diagnostic and Statistical Manual of Mental Disorders* (DSM-III) published by the American Psychosocial Association (Crocq & Crocq, 2000). The term *PTSD* is associated with the aftermath or legacy of the Vietnam War. Common references to soldiers struggling during or after earlier conflicts were *shell shock, war neurosis,* and *combat exhaustion.* Fortunately, along with a more appropriate name, time brought an improved understanding of the condition, such as it not being an inherent individual weakness (traumatic neurosis) but rather an etiological agent outside the individual. The decade of the 1980s definitely brought in a new way of thinking about post-traumatic stress, whether associated with combat, physical abuse, car accident, or some other major life event.

The challenges of PTSD can be daunting and leave you feeling completely helpless. As well, many people with post-traumatic stress also have incurred a head injury, which often interacts with PTSD compounding the struggle. The good news is, there are a number of ways in which people are being helped. First and foremost, counselors trained in the treatment of PTSD are helping through what they call cognitive behavioral therapy. This is a tried-and-true process whereby people with PTSD understand and change how they think about their trauma and its aftermath. It's a way to bring about clarity to toxic thoughts that often make symptoms more intense. Through cognitive restructuring, exposure therapy, and the management of specific symptoms, patients are being helped all over the world.

The great outdoors can help to improve overall stress levels as part of a holistic approach to healing. Bielinis et al. (2019) stated, "The positive effect [the forest has] on the mental health and well being of those suffering from post-traumatic stress disorder or experiencing stress has been proven" (p. 1). Spending time in the forest, according to the authors, is any activity in a forest environment as a means to refresh and improve health. Forest therapy, as it is also called, is a means whereby the great outdoors helps individuals cope with anxiety, depression, and a host of other challenges. Studies that include outdoors therapy, specifically related to war veterans diagnosed with PTSD, have also been shown to reduce stress for these veterans (Poulsen et al., 2016). Poulson et al. found that veterans were still using nature as a stress reducer one year after the study was complete.

As well, Pálsdóttir et al. (2017) state, "Natural environments can have a positive impact on human health and well being, restore cognitive functions, improve self-reported health, and facilitate stress restoration" (p. 1). In my own life, I've found that routinely taking long walks outdoors does improve my overall perspective and, ultimately, my health. The bottom line is that the person suffering from PTSD and/or PCS should find what works best for them. If possible, they should push through symptoms and embrace the beauty that is all about them. This can take time, but the payoff is a more fulfilled life and more meaningful time with family and friends.

For the person suffering from PTSD, it's as though they were back on the battlefield, standing near their abuser, or about to be T-boned. It's an emotional wrenching situated somewhere in the chasm between virtual reality and truth. The flashbacks, distressful thoughts, anxiety, depression, and nightmares are excruciating, even leading some to commit suicide. No one should endure this type of pain alone or indefinitely. PTSD affects millions of people around the world, bringing overwhelming feelings of hopelessness and fear. If you or someone in your family is living with PTSD, reach out for help. Whether through a counselor trained in treating PTSD, spending time in the great outdoors, increasing an exercise regimen, volunteering to help others in need, or all of the above, it is possible to return your soul to a place of peace.

8

Finding Your Eden

"Hope deferred makes the heart sick, but a dream fulfilled is a tree of life," exclaims King Solomon (Proverbs 13:12, NLT). People who've sustained a TBI hope for complete healing or, at least, measurable improvement. They long that their PCS symptoms will fly away, never to light upon them again. Like a hurricane slamming into the coastlands, leaving its wake of destruction, post-concussion symptoms are unpredictable both in their timing and intensity. There is no rhyme or reason as the pain and pressure bring about a sense of hopelessness. And where is Eden during these most challenging of times? Where does the head-injured person turn when answers slip farther and farther away?

Kindra and I found a little town in northern Texas, not far from the big city of Dallas. Farmersville had a population of just over 3,000 and some of the friendliest people we'd ever met. The townsfolk were proud of their community and happy to discuss its historic Onion Shed and famous former resident Audie Murphy. Known as the most decorated US soldier, Murphy came home to a hero's welcome on July 16, 1945. I loved listening to the locals share about their town with such enthusiasm and pride. And as we crossed the brick-laden streets of the town square, I was inspired to think about Eden one more

10.4324/9781003216056-8

time. I pondered the contrast between our experience in the beautiful Utah mountain town and my accident shortly thereafter.

What was the purpose of a debilitating head injury as we were on the precipice of something exciting and new? Just prior to the accident, my wife and I strolled Eden as a gentle breeze made its way through the hill country and brushed against our skin, rounding a sense of optimism and hope. I thought deeply about Eden and the accident as we entered another historic building to order two specialty coffees again. The coffee house 12 Stories Coffee represented Farmersville very well with its nod to the modern world set in the confines of a history-laden building. I wondered how many locals had crossed its vestibule over the years ordering up their own coffee or other special delights. We ordered lattes because we loved the special touch of a good barista.

I stood quietly as the barista handed over our lattes with perfect white hearts resting peacefully on the surface. Something very special was happening at that moment, but I didn't quite understand it at first. It was a surreal experience and indescribably beautiful. The feeling was overwhelming as I stood there, simply gazing into the cup. After all this time since the accident, which had changed my life in so many ways, had I finally found Eden? It was as though the sun had finally begun to rise, warming my face after a very long and cold night. My eyes became misty at the new revelation. Yes, I found Eden; more precisely, we had found Eden. At that very moment in time, in a little town called Farmersville, the search was finally over. There she was in all her glory, Eden, and with her life-altering message of hope.

Why was the meaning not clear before visiting that little Farmersville coffee shop? Why didn't I understand that Eden wasn't a physical location but a place in the heart? It was a profound message hidden from me for a very long time. Certainly, I had an idea that Eden was more than a physical place, but the renewing of my spirit never came until that moment. Hopelessness and despair had reigned in my heart, but now I could see more clearly. Eden was there all the time, but I wasn't emotionally ready to accept her message. The post-concussion symptoms had ruled everything about me, from my relationships, ability to work, and even my ability to communicate. And now, after a long season of struggle, it was time to overcome.

Eden became my symbol of hope. The barista in Eden, who forgot to lock the front door all those months ago, welcomed us in with a warm smile and lattes on the house. She didn't top the drinks with leafy designs or rosette patterns but with the heart-shaped symbol of love. And now, it was the same in Farmersville, a heart-shaped representation of love. It was a message of hopefulness that I was finally ready to embrace. My long-awaited epiphany didn't mean an end to the headaches, pressure, disorientation, or any other of the post-concussion symptoms but an end to the struggling of my soul. I could now move forward with an attitude of hopefulness supported by a heart of love. It was finally my turn for transformation, and I was ready.

If you or a loved one has sustained a head injury, the "winds" are definitely pressing hard against you. No doubt about it. Use those winds to push your vessel along at an even greater speed. The contrast, if you do nothing at all to properly adjust your life to the new circumstance, is that your vessel may sink. What will your catalyst for change be? When will you adjust your sails to the challenges of a brain injury? This is not an easy process, especially for those individuals with more severe injuries. But if the sails can be adjusted, they should be. For me, "changing of the sails" happened in an unassuming small-town coffee house.

Using HOPEFUL as an acronym, the following provides a proactive approach for the person suffering from TBI and PCS. This roadmap will not replace the important guidance of an excellent counselor. Rather, it provides additional support while recognizing and honoring the work of healthcare professionals. Having an attitude of hopefulness, or simply being hopeful, can help foster a sense of optimism for the person with TBI. Let your story unfold as a masterpiece blessing your family, friends, and others who cross your path. Let your testimony be the magnum opus inspiring others to succeed in the face of great odds. Each letter of the acronym below represents a different aspect of hopefulness, drawing you closer to the honorable objective of inner healing and peace.

HOPEFUL

Honor Yourself: Honoring oneself rubs the grain for many of us who were raised to honor others but with a heart of humility. "You must love yourself first before you can properly love others" is a common vernacular and important for the person dealing with PCS. However, it's difficult to honor yourself when your head hurts and you can't string a coherent sentence together. But honoring yourself goes beyond a feeling or emotion. It's an abiding commitment from your core that no matter how you feel mentally, physically, or emotionally, you will carry on with the same distinctive principles that characterized you before the injury.

Margarita Tartakovsky (2016) emphasizes the importance of not only honoring ourselves but also accepting everything about ourselves, including imperfections—in other words, embracing the disappointments as part of a tapestry in our personal journey. That's not to say we stop growing in our knowledge, physicality, and spiritual dimensions, but we are at peace with who we are in the process. I came to know someone many years ago who was an incredible pianist. I was enraptured as she played the world-renowned piece that Hector Berlioz described as a "lamentation" in Beethoven's *Moonlight Sonata* (first movement). It was as though she and the music were one as she swayed with its slow and steady progression. The saddest day came when she decided to stop playing. Her piano sat quietly until she returned to her hometown on the south coast of England.

Amelia wanted desperately to return to her homeland, but circumstances prevented her from doing so. She described her town as a magical place with the purest seawater anywhere. She talked endlessly about its pine forest landscapes and crisp, breathable air, a catalyst for so many creative geniuses in the area. I loved our conversations but missed hearing her play. Before she ultimately found her way home, she explained to me that she would play again, but not till her feet stepped on English soil. It wasn't about England or the United States; it was about a deep longing for home. But I always felt that since she learned to play while growing up in England, maybe playing again would take her back, if only in her remembering?

Maybe under similar circumstances, I, too, may have stopped the music. I know what it's like to be away from your homeland and yearn deeply for your family, friends, and familiar surroundings. And for Amelia, even the sounds of the crashing ocean played their own music, and she longed for those sounds. The natural environment in Amelia's homeland called out to her many times while she was growing up. It was her inspiration for improving her craft from childhood into her early adult years. And now that her inspiration was gone, so was her playing. She was one of those very special people that step into your life for just a brief moment of time yet leave an indelible impression.

Someday, my wife and I will travel to the south coast of England to see if we can find Amelia. I would love to hear her play once again. It was through my brief friendship with her that I learned a life lesson about perspective. I'm not saying that Amelia was wrong to stop playing while she was in the States. Not at all. However, it takes several years to learn an instrument well, especially the piano. She spent her learning years while growing up in England. Maybe playing her music abroad could have taken her back in some sense? Again, I'm not saying Amelia was "wrong," only that life challenges have more than one perspective.

Before my brain injury, I used to teach business courses at a local college. One of the courses I taught, Business Ethics, provided opportunities for discussion among my students. As the teacher, I tried to direct the students toward meaningful conversations about real-life scenarios or dilemmas. In one example, I asked students to think about a scenario where local prisoners were brought outside the prison grounds once per week. In a cohort of 20, they were taken to pick up garbage along the local highway.

As they were working, a car passed with a driver and passenger. The passenger commented to the driver, "It's sad enough that they have to be locked up in prison. Now they are paraded in front of the entire world for everyone to see. How embarrassing!"

Then a second vehicle passed with a driver and passenger. The passenger in that vehicle had a different perspective: "I can't imagine being locked up in jail, day in and day out. It's so wonderful the guards let them out for sunshine once in a while!"

The prisoner example demonstrates that there is always more than one perspective. Without question, TBI can bring challenges that are overwhelming. However, how one responds to the challenge is up to the individual. In essence, it's about honoring the self. There was a time in my own journey that I let the post-concussion symptoms overwhelm me. I allowed room for the darkness, making me feel hopeless, helpless, and depressed. In spite of the off-and-on symptoms, I needed a new perspective to return to my true identity. I like Chip Gains's perspective on this. While referring to his good friend, Gabe Grunewald, who was an American professional middle-distance runner, he stated, "There is never a situation so dark that light cannot shine, never a scenario so bleak that hope can't pull us through." Chip was referring to Gabe's unyielding optimism through her cancer treatments and eventual passing. Through all her suffering, Gabe became an inspiration to others who were suffering around the world, including me. Gabe honored others by honoring herself.

Occupy: Being *in the moment* rather than allowing oneself to *mentally drift* during conversations is important for the person with TBI. One of many ways to reinspire your listening, or being in the moment, is to be intentional about getting outdoors. With the forests of Burleigh Heads National Park in Australia as the backdrop, Qiu et al. (2021) wanted to know if "listening to the forests" or what makes natural sounds "[would] renew and re-energize people, especially in the face of significant stressors" (p. 1). The researchers were able to link improvements in mental health to nature experiences. While listening to the forest would be a wonderful idea for the head-injured person, the juxtaposition is that listening, or being in the moment, is very important.

Unless you are exhausted and needing rest, push against your mental drift. It's an opportunity for your brain to exercise, grow, stimulate, and work the neurotransmitters. When you engage in conversation, especially one requiring deeper levels of thought, neurons release neurotransmitters, or electrical signals, in neighboring neurons. The electrical signals cultivate like a wave to thousands of neurons, which ultimately leads to thought formation. While it's impossible to completely shut down your brain, even when you feel mentally adrift, it's best that you *practice* pushing your brain like the muscle it is. Over time, become an athlete of sorts and exercise that muscle more and more through various forms of stimulation.

Another problem I developed after my brain injury was stumbling on my words. Speech therapists call this word finding. It's frustrating while talking with someone to find my words coming out garbled and difficult to understand. There are ways to reduce this problem, such as allowing extra time before speaking, talking more slowly, using shorter sentences, and rehearsing what you want to say in advance. However, the main point I want to make relates to the dynamics within a back-and-forth conversation, which I've noticed can bring about an increased stumbling of words.

Don't be afraid to dialogue with someone while you're having symptoms. The goal is to exercise your mind, to stimulate those neurons. If I'm being completely honest, I struggle in this area and sometimes avoid conversations while symptomatic, especially with a colleague. However, if I'm garbling my words while talking with my spouse, it gives me an opportunity to exercise those neurons in hopes of improving in the long term. My goal is to stay in the moment as much as possible, embracing a holistic approach to my recovery. The idea is to "occupy" or stay present. Don't allow yourself to mentally drift. Stay focused. Stay in the moment as much as possible. Exercise your brain. In doing these things, you'll be honoring yourself and those around you. As well, you will help to maintain a positive attitude of hopefulness.

Participate: In addition to staying in the moment, find a task that will also keep your brain exercised and focused. One of the best ways to get your brain charged and back on track is through creativity. What is your gift? What is it that you were passionate about before your injury? Are you still doing those things? Did you write beautiful music or play an instrument? I play a musical instrument, but I have never played at Amelia's level. Creativity is not about a particular level of proficiency. It's about the process of creating and how your brain interacts with that process.

The idea that creative expression has a positive effect on healing has been around for a long time. Music engagement, in particular, can have a profound effect on healing in the area of anxiety, even helping to bring about a restoration of emotional balance (Stuckey & Nobel, 2010). It's my belief that the creative process, whether through the composition of music or the building of an ornate armoire, can help in the healing process. In their work, Nathan and Mirviss (1998) state, "[O]ur senses, bodies, thoughts, and feelings, are stimulated through using creative arts." The complex mind-body connection has been discussed and researched more frequently in recent years as counselors seek best practices and methodologies in treating various forms of injury and illness. In fact, Perryman et al. state, "Understanding the mind-body connection has become increasingly important for counselors in searching for effective strategies to affect physical and psychological well-being" (p. 83).

With me as an example, my particular creative bent falls more toward writing than playing a musical instrument. Although both would have some benefit in my healing, my preference at this point in my life is to write. In fact, I have noticed that as I've dedicated more time to my writing recently, my symptoms have been less severe and have not lasted as long. I'm certainly not claiming a "smoking gun" in the reduction of symptoms; I'm only sharing my recent experience. Like many individuals who suffer from PCS, there are times when my symptoms are so intense; I wouldn't be able to engage in any type of creative endeavor. But if you can get creative when the symptoms are less severe, it might be helpful for your overall prognosis. Use your creativity as a launching board to a more hopeful and optimistic future.

Educate: When my accident happened, we knew almost nothing about head injuries or PCS. However, after stumbling on my words just a few hours after the accident, we began to realize the importance of learning everything we could about head trauma. Becoming adept in a matter, especially related to an accident or illness, can be time-consuming but worth every minute. Learning all you can about your specific injury empowers you to make good decisions as you move forward.

One reliable organization is the UK-based non-profit organization, Headway: The Brain Injury Association (Headway.org.uk). Their website provides supportive information on a wide range of issues and even a confidential helpline for head-injured individuals or their family members. Other organizations, such as the Brain Trauma Foundation, translate neuroscience into effective solutions. This organization advises medical professionals on best practice guidelines related to the latest research. Extra caution should be taken if visiting non-professional pages, such as personal blog sites where good information might be mixed with personal, non-research-based opinion.

To educate oneself on a particular matter is to move from the shadows of mere curiosity to the light of discernment. For the person with persistent post-concussion symptoms, entering that "light" requires a significant commitment to the learning process and what that entails. Learning all you can about your specific head injury and post-concussion symptoms in general will help you be more concise with your family doctor, neurologist, and other medical specialists. In essence, a better understanding of your condition helps you to become a better advocate for yourself. Help your doctor help you. Once you've educated yourself on the basics of PCS, you might ask your doctor these additional questions:

- What should I do if new symptoms develop?
- What are my treatment options?
- Are there potential side effects for the treatment?
- Are there alternative treatments available?
- What about additional diagnostic tests for my head injury?
- Am I a candidate for enrolling in a neurological clinic?

Be your own best advocate on your healing journey by conducting meaningful research and becoming a proactive member of your healthcare team.

Fulfill: Living a fulfilled life should always be the objective, accident or not. Because post-concussion symptoms can be overwhelming, even ushering the injured person to some very dark places, more reason to seek out those important interests you had before the accident. If you've been able to continue your passions after the head injury, you are doing very well. Many people struggle to break free from their "hiding place." It's a lonely way of life that's difficult to describe, let alone understand. The pain and pressure associated with a head injury can cause one to shut down, even become withdrawn from other people. It's almost like all four engines have failed on a large jetliner, leaving an eerie quiet and the pilot desperately looking for a place to land.

Before my accident, I enjoyed the company of others; I was seen as outgoing and a people person. I felt comfortable in groups and working alongside others at the jobsite. I had a wide range of friends and knew a lot of people. In fact, as an in-class college instructor, I interacted with large groups of people almost daily. I even landed on the "Extraversion" (E) side of the Myers-Briggs personality test. However, after my accident, I became more of an introvert, preferring instead to be alone and out of the limelight. I was increasingly detached and wondering where the old me might have gone. I didn't want to go outside the home and struggled to communicate with my family. When I did venture out into the world, I avoided conversation and even avoided eye contact as much as possible. More and more, I allowed the darkness to overpower me as I spent countless hours at home and alone.

In one of her secret missions to break me out of my shell, Kindra invited me to the historic Georgetown Square. The town square was one of my favorite places in the world, and I really wanted to go. But as usual, I declined the invitation using my head pain as one of many reasons. Grace Ononiwune, one of Britain's top lawyers, would have been proud as I offered up a defense that included every symptom and the possibility of rain later that afternoon. Kindra's response was classic—she smiled, retrieved her car keys, and said she'd meet me outside.

The Georgetown Square was bustling with people as we passed through on our way to a nearby parking lot. We brought our son's Alaskan Klee Kai, which looks exactly like a miniature husky. Akaira is the same dog who accompanied us when we happened upon a rattlesnake while out strolling a few months earlier. Akaira has a great personality, is highly sociable, and is always up for a walk. We made our way to a little antique shop near the square with an assortment of collectibles, from stained glass to antique furniture. Kindra disappeared into the store as I made myself comfortable on an outdoor bench. The bench seemed like a good place to "hide" since my symptoms were at the higher end of the ten scale, and I didn't want to talk with anyone.

My plan for quiet repose didn't work out. It seemed that every visitor to Georgetown Square noticed Akaira and wanted to stop at the bench. I was increasingly uncomfortable as more people continued showing up. I tried my best to be polite but kept looking to see if Kindra might be coming out soon. All kinds of people dropped by the bench. People who were alone stopped by. There were young people, old people, and every age in between. Then, over the course of several minutes, something miraculous happened. Even though my symptoms were intense, my heart began to soften. I found myself smiling and engaging in conversations. Everyone was so kind. They were smiling, laughing, and genuinely at the moment. These strangers at

Georgetown Square were drawing me out of my dark shell and back to my former self.

Kindra's insistence that I join her that day actually paid big dividends. I learned in one setting that my symptoms could not control my destiny. I pushed myself through the pain and increased my outings over the next several months. The more I stepped out, symptoms or not, the more confidence I gained in my own ability to even socialize with strangers. There is still the great temptation to stay at home, accept the darkness, and let life pass on by. However, pushing through the darkness and setting a new path is entirely possible. If you are stuck in the nether regions, feeling unsociable, confined, and confused, consider reaching out to your loved one or counselor for guidance. In my case, it turns out that both my spouse and professional counselor were correct. I could get to the light, but I needed a little push.

Undo: There are many different causes for head injuries, both traumatic (motor vehicle accidents, falls, violence, military attack, etc.) and non-traumatic (stroke, tumors, lack of oxygen, etc.), that can bring about a great deal of trepidation for the injured person. An all-too-common response following a head injury is fear that the event will happen again. It's important to begin to let go of false assumptions, such as an "inevitable" future car crash. Undo these fears as part of your healing journey returning to a life of normalcy. Keep in mind, however, that the undoing process might be time-consuming and require the help of a professional counselor. In the highly acclaimed American film *What About Bob*, Bob (Bill Murray) determined near the end of the film that his counselor, Dr. Leo Marvin (Richard Dreyfuss), wanted him to "untie his knots." He was partly speaking to his own false assumptions.

If you've allowed fear to grip your life because of a head injury, consider seeking counsel from a professional. I have always been an advocate for good counseling but avoided talking to a professional after my accident. This probably had more to do with my attitude of self-sufficiency rather than anything else. Fortunately, I eventually reached out to a counselor trained in TBI and PCS. She was incredibly helpful from a professional standpoint and was a good listener. I was impressed with her balance of thoughtful advice, active listening, and true empathy. She cared about my struggles and wanted to provide meaningful direction to help me progress. If you are struggling after your accident, maybe it's time to undo any false assumptions holding you back. Perhaps this important step can be accomplished through the help of an excellent counselor trained in your specific type of injury.

Love: John Muir, the Scottish-American naturalist and environmental philosopher, states, "The mountains are calling and I must go." In my travels, I've heard the mountains call out to me, but I never truly listened until after my accident. The most difficult events in life are that way; they bring about a higher understanding and appreciation of those things around us. This is what the runner Sandra Duran meant when she stated, "The little things appear that may have otherwise been just a blur." It's taking time to slow down and truly appreciate the beauty that is all about you. It's in that quiet place that the colors become more vibrant, the sounds more clear, smells more fragrant, and the touch more meaningful.

Being hopeful, as the acronym conveys, is very important to your long-term success and overall health. PCS is crafty and does not have your best interest in mind. It wants nothing less than the entirety of your life. Don't let the symptoms win. Be proactive by maintaining a heart of hopefulness against all the many challenges associated with your head injury. It can be a herculean struggle that will take your full attention. You can be victorious, but it will take a commitment on your part. It will require placing your house in order and staying committed to your own healing journey. In the process, consider the time-honored metaphor of the building and how it can relate to your own situation.

The soundness of a building is dependent on its foundation. Contractors often refer to the foundation of a building as the most important component because of its load-bearing capabilities and capacity to anchor a structure from heavy winds and other natural forces. For the person suffering from PCS, there should be a solid starting point on which all other things rely. Your entire outlook/worldview should be built upon a foundation on which you can depend. Even when the harsh winds of adversity press against you, and the symptoms seem more than you can bear, your building will stand because you have a deep-rooted commitment to its stability. In other words, at your core, there should be something so exceptional that it informs everything else.

Before the modern era, architects relied on something at least as significant (if not more) than the foundation of a building. Not having the conveniences of later technologies, builders laid a cornerstone and used it as a reference point for other corners of the building as well as keeping the walls straight. In fact, the total weight of a structure depended on the cornerstone for its integrity. If removed, the building would collapse. The cornerstone gave the building its strength, character, and exact position in the world. I have a friend who works in the building industry. He loves history, especially related to the study of architecture and how it has evolved over the centuries and across many different cultures. He once referred to the cornerstones of yesteryear as the backbone or heart of a building.

What will be your cornerstone? What is it that you can look to for strength when your days are at their worst? Many people living through the debilitating symptoms of PCS feel hopeless, as though their lives no longer had meaning.

They become tired and overcome by their symptoms, eventually unwilling to reach out for help or a stronger perspective. In my own journey, I have experienced deep hopelessness, helplessness, anxiety, and depression. I also had most of the other symptoms of PCS. My post-accident self did not represent the real me. Not by a long shot. Before the accident, I was outgoing and loved being with other people. I was what the internationally acclaimed Myers and Briggs Foundation would call an extraverted personality.

It was as though the brain injury had changed my core self as I allowed the symptoms to become my cornerstone and inform everything about me. No longer did I want to spend time with others, not even my family. Completely shutting down, I felt more comfortable in a darkened room, sometimes staring at the wall. It was a challenge to string cohesive thoughts together, let alone a meaningful and loving conversation with others. But my spouse would not let me sink to nothingness. She was the one who became my foundation. It was her love and support that helped me embrace hope. If it weren't for her tenacity, I would not have recognized a life lesson that came full circle at a small coffee shop in Farmersville.

Eleanor Farjeon was born in Strand, London, in 1881. She was an influential author of poetry, children's stories, plays, history, and satire. She won many awards and came from a family of writers and composers. In fact, she penned one of my all-time favorite poems that I first loved way back in elementary school. Its words encapsulate my entire long journey since the accident. The village of Alfriston in East Sussex originally inspired the song, but it has since appeared in many places as a way to give thanks and recognition for each day. The song was also made popular by the English pop musician and folk singer Cat Stevens. "Morning Has Broken" has become my anthem for a new day far beyond the restless seas of PCS:

> Morning has broken,
> Like the first morning,
> Blackbird has spoken
> Like the first bird;
> Praise for the singing,
> Praise for the morning,
> Praise for them springing
> Fresh from the word.
>
> Sweet the rain's new fall,
> Sunlit from heaven,
> Like the first dewfall
> On the first grass;
> Praise for the sweetness,
> Of the wet garden,
> Sprung in completeness
> Where His feet pass.
>
> Mine is the sunlight,
> Mine is the morning,
> Born of the one light

Eden saw play;
Praise with elation,
Praise every morning
God's re-creation
Of the new day.

9

Coping Strategies for Psychological Effects of Brain Injury

Psychological reactions to TBI are varied and complex. In my clinical practice, TBI survivors and their families present the most with depression, anxiety, and PTSD. Dr. Michael Arthur brilliantly describes his own struggles with these mental health issues. Sadly, depression and anxiety are the most frequently diagnosed mood disorders in TBI survivors (Collins et al., 2012). These emotional disturbances following TBI may be due to "a disruption of affective brain systems and/or the stress of adjustment to post-injury environmental demands" (Rush et al., 2006). Jorge (2008) finds that mood disturbances had a large impact on family relationships, social integration, and return to productive activity. He also stated the mood disturbances affected caregivers and TBI survivors and accounted for a significant part of the disability resulting in TBI of any severity. Douglas and Spellacy (2000) documented the prevalence of depression and anxiety was similar for primary caregivers of TBI survivors. They continue that half of the survivors studied reported significant levels of depression that did not dissipate over time. Alternative treatments recommended for caregivers and survivors were cognitive behavioral therapy, education, family therapy, and support groups (Marsh et al., 2002). Social

10.4324/9781003216056-9

support in the form of community, social network, and intimate and confiding relationships met the long-term needs of adults with TBI and their caregivers (Douglas & Spellacy, 2000).

Major Depressive Disorder

Although there is a wide variation in the prevalence of major depressive disorder, most recent studies estimate that between 45–53% of individuals with complicated mild to severe TBI experience a depressive episode in the first year of the injury. The most conservative estimates place TBI survivors at higher risk for developing depression than the general population. Jones and Jorge report that 29.4% of TBI survivors experience depression during the first year post-injury (Jones & Jorge, 2019). In 2009, Hawthorne and coworkers concluded that TBI survivors

> experienced worse general health, elevated probabilities of depression, social isolation and worse labor force participation rates . . . unless treatment includes targeting services at those areas of life identified in this and other studies, limited outcomes can be expected.

The prevalence and negative impact of depression on psychosocial functioning, quality of life, and increased suicidal ideation highlight the need for accurate assessment and effective treatment (Ashman et al., 2014). Stress and allostatic load, a concept referring to the long-lasting effects of persistently activated stress reactions, have been linked to the development of depression post-TBI (McIntyre et al., 2020). Therefore, early detection of those at risk for post-traumatic depression and the development of effective prevention and treatment could improve the long-term outcomes for TBI survivors (Juengst et al., 2015). Specific to brain injury, depression can be caused by damage to the frontal, subcortical, and limbic areas of the brain. There can be a steady increase in onset up until two to three years post-injury due to the increased awareness of the injury and its accompanying deficits, such as the loss of freedom and independence, limitations in activity, loss of self, impaired ability to think and reason, and loss of social network. In this case, depression can be considered a part of the recovery process. Awareness often creates feelings of despondency and anxiousness. The moods of despondency may come and go over days, weeks, or months. Additionally, family members may notice the client has become depressed after an initial improvement in their recovery. Educating the family that a depressive reaction is common helps normalize the experience as a part of the recovery process. Gronwall et al. (1998) state that recognizing these mood disturbances as a normal response allows the rehabilitation to proceed in a positive manner.

According to the fifth edition of the *Diagnostic and Statistical Manual of Mental Disorders* (DSM-V), the criterion for major depressive disorder is the presence of a depressed mood or loss of interest for at least two weeks. Additionally, the individual may experience a combination of weight changes, sleep problems (insomnia or hypersomnia), slowed movement, fatigue or loss of energy, feeling worthless and guilty, diminished ability to think or make decisions, and recurrent thoughts of death (DSM-V, 2013). Diagnosing major depressive disorder after TBI can be challenging. Several of the symptoms of depression mimic the sequelae of TBI. For example, both TBI and depression exhibit fatigue, low mood, cognitive deficits, and sleep disturbance. Mood changes for depression include sadness, tearfulness, agitation, and irritability. Examples of behavior changes are psychomotor agitation or retardation, social withdrawal, poor hygiene, and lack of motivation. Common cognitive symptoms are helplessness, hopelessness, self-criticism, indecisiveness, and loss of interest. To determine the source as an emotional disturbance versus the direct result of a brain injury, the clinician must obtain a thorough history with the client and (if possible) the family. Involvement of family is important because the awareness and recall of the client may be impaired. For example, the family member may report that the loved one sits and cries daily, but the survivor may report feeling "a little sad." Other issues, such as pseudobulbar affect (PBA), contribute to miscommunication because the survivor suddenly expresses laughter or crying without reason. The sudden mood changes are difficult to navigate when the expression is opposite of how the survivor is actually feeling. The inability to express the feeling accurately can be a common occurrence, especially in the early stages of brain injury. In short, TBI survivors who seek treatment for depression vary in their ability to acknowledge their depressive emotions and behaviors accurately (Ruff & Jamora, 2008).

Coping Strategies

The goal of managing depression is reducing and/or eliminating the symptoms. The first line of defense with any mental health issue is to schedule a physical with their primary doctor to rule out any medical issues that may present as depression or contribute to depression. Sometimes medication is prescribed on a short-term to long-term basis. Of course, it is preferable to work with a physician who is familiar with mental health and TBI diagnoses.

Social support makes a significant impact in lowering depression. Previous research demonstrated that the lack of social contact remained a permanent long-term outcome for TBI survivors. Tomberg et al. (2005) study a group of TBI survivors in Estonia, a post-socialist country. The study demonstrated that the availability of potential supporters helped alleviate the effects of stress and offered positive adjustment and appropriate problem solving for TBI survivors. The presence of individuals who were able to consistently provide care, help, trust, and emotional support remained essential for long-term rehabilitation. Support mainly came from family members, while the number of non-relatives among supporters was significantly lower. The study identified that a poorer support system was indicative of an inadequate or malfunctioning supporters' network that did not correspond to the individual's needs. The quality of support relationships made more difference than the number of supporters. One study showed that 31% of TBI survivors had no friends outside of their family (Hoofien et al., 2001). Several studies documented the difficulties TBI survivors had in maintaining social function. Loss of social contact, difficulty making new friends, and misinterpretation of social cues characterized poor functioning. Understanding this, Hope After Brain Injury offers a monthly support group for brain injury survivors and family members. They also host quarterly dinner and movie night in which they rent a movie theater that provides dinner, popcorn, and a movie. They have found this to be a well-attended event that helps create community and social support with others who have common challenges.

Self-care is essential for TBI survivors and their families. Along with patience and understanding, self-care is a consistent need for successful recovery. Exercise, taking vitamins, and journaling are the three recommendations I offer to each client in the brain injury journey. Exercise is simply movement. Planned movement is scheduling a time to walk, run, practice yoga, golf, bike, or clean house. Begin with the safest movement and gradually build to a sustained pace. A moderate increase in intensity and length of time can be an ongoing goal. Taking vitamins contribute to overall health. Vitamin D is a favorite recommendation. As a natural sun supplement, studies have shown that vitamin D can improve brain health. Spending at least 20 minutes outside in the sun or even if it is overcast helps one breathe, gain perspective, and reset. Journaling offers two advantages. The first is simply expression. Writing down one's thoughts helps relieve the brain of trying to remember and gives the writer a safe outlet to express himself. One TBI survivor reported that she wrote all of her "firsts" since waking from the coma—the first time she brushed her hair, the first time she drove, and the first speaking engagement were some of her entries. Journaling everyday events also helps one document progress. With short-term memory loss, this is a huge help to TBI survivors. The second advantage is exploration. Often one comes to understand a problem or an issue in the process of writing. It is not uncommon for the writer to recognize a clear solution once the issue is thought out through the writing exercise. The creativity of writing also strengthens the brain and helps build the neuropathways for recovery. The lasting benefit is the gain of insight and awareness.

Generalized Anxiety Disorder

According to the DSM-V, generalized anxiety disorder (GAD) is a part of the anxiety disorders spectrum. Anxiety, along with depression, is commonly diagnosed with

TBI survivors and family members. Studies document that the prevalence of anxiety in this population ranges between 10 and 33% (Albrecht et al., 2017). GAD is characterized by at least six months of excessive worry and anxiety. The DSM-V (2013) describes the condition whereby one struggles to control worry and experiences significant distress in social, occupational, and family functioning. In addition, the person may experience a combination of symptoms, such as restlessness, easily fatigued, irritability, difficulty concentrating, and/or sleep disturbance. For an accurate diagnosis, it is necessary to assess the presence of a relationship between the onset, exacerbation, or remission of the general medical condition and the anxiety symptoms. Depression and anxiety are associated with the TBI survivor's loss of independence, loss of self, and loss related to a prior level of high functioning. Rudi Coetzer (2018) states that one of the psychological concepts of GAD relevant to TBI survivors is the issue of control. The cognitive impairments contribute to a "reduced ability to control the environments or to solve problems that may appear straightforward or even trivial to deal with in the past" (Coetzer, 2018). Additionally, some of the physical symptoms of brain injury, such as dizziness, tremors, and sleep disturbance, may contribute to anxiety. Coetzer (2018) differentiates the symptoms that are specific to TBI but not necessarily GAD. These include (1) realistic worries about the future in response to TBI, (2) fatigue and poor concentration, and (3) irritability. As with depression, the symptoms of anxiety can mimic the deficits of TBI. Keen assessment is imperative to proper diagnosis and treatment.

Coping Strategies

The key to managing anxiety is reducing its symptoms. One of the main strategies recommended is diaphragmic breathing. Sighing is often a signal that one is not breathing through one's diaphragm. It's as though the body is trying to catch its breath. Proper, deep breathing begins with inhaling through the nose and exhaling through the mouth. Inhaling through the mouth activates the sympathetic nervous system, thereby creating a fight-or-flight response. So instead of alleviating anxiety, inhaling through your mouth activates anxiety. Tactical breathing, also called box or square breathing, is a technique initially used for the military but has found a helpful place in the civilian population. The four-step process is this: (1) inhale through the nose to the count of four, (2) hold one's breath to the count of four, (3) exhale through the mouth to the count of four, and (4) hold one's breath to the count of four. This can be practiced in almost all settings, from sitting at a traffic light to participating in a board meeting. Practicing tactical breathing when not anxious helps create the habit that one can apply in an anxious situation.

Other coping strategies include relaxation, biofeedback, visual imagery, and cognitive restructuring (Coetzer, 2018). Progressive relaxation in which one tightens and releases muscle groups from the top of the head to the bottom of the feet is helpful. Biofeedback is a process of gaining an understanding of the body's response to stimulus and using specialized technology to thereby relieve the stimulus or anxiety. Typically, biofeedback is a specialty practiced by a certified biofeedback therapist. Guided imagery is creating mental images of calming scenes or relaxing places where the person may "travel" to when anxious. Cognitive restructuring requires the person to recognize the anxiety-provoking thoughts and replacing them with rational thoughts. In my practice, we discuss the what-if spiral. Asking "What if this happens?" or "What if that happens?" tends to increase fear and anxiety.

My recommendation is to replace the what-if with what's true. What's true is that, for example, my family member is safe, my mother knows who to contact in an emergency, and so on. Concentrating on what is true at the moment helps anchor the person and decrease anxiety. Pacing is another suggestion made in my practice. Clients often will hear me recommend, "Add grace to your pace." Often TBI survivors who were go-getters before the injury want to recover at a go-getter pace. However, the brain doesn't accommodate that speed. While it is creating new neuropathways, it is advisable for the survivor to be gentle with himself. Manageable pacing decreases anxiety, improves functionality, reduces mistakes, and reduces fatigue.

Ponsford (2013) recommend coping strategies, such as problem-solving, developing a positive outlook, and utilizing humor as helpful to reduce anxiety. Reassurance that the client is not going crazy or losing their minds is an important strategy as well, especially for chronic anxiety (Ponsford, 2013). Recognizing the client's worries and allowing them to voice those worries is a significant step toward understanding the underlying issues that fuel their anxiety. Additionally, it is imperative to assist the client toward hopeful outcomes. When working with TBI survivors who struggle with anxiety, it is restorative to help the client pursue "personally salient goals" (Coetzer, 2018). Ponsford (2013) recommends distraction and cognitive restructuring as a means to gain control over the thoughts that accompany anxiety. Anchoring oneself is another recommendation to stave off accelerated anxiety. Another term for that is grounding. It is a technique whereby one focuses on what is seen, heard, smelled, and felt, being mindful of the minute instead of fearing the future. With TBI survivors, anxiety can stem from sensory overload.

Environmental factors such as bright lights, music, loud voices, cross-talking, and noises from multiple sources can and will overload a TBI survivor. Stepping away and excusing oneself from the environment will help reduce the anxiety and offer a peaceful, calm respite.

Post-Traumatic Stress Disorder

PTSD has been widely studied since World War I. The condition survived several names, such as shell shock, battle or combat fatigue, and stress syndrome. PTSD is considered one of the trauma- and stressor-related disorders in the DSM-V. To be diagnosed with PTSD, one must have been exposed to actual or threatened death, serious injury, or sexual violence by either experiencing the trauma directly, witnessing the trauma, or learning that a traumatic event happened to a family member or close friend. Additionally, the person experiences a combination of the following: recurrent or intrusive memories, distressing dreams, flashbacks, aversive reaction to triggering events, avoidance of stimuli associated with the trauma, inability to remember important aspects of the trauma, irritability, hypervigilance, exaggerated startle response, self-destructive behavior, feeling detached or negative emotional state, inability to experience positive emotion, and sleep disturbance (DSM-V, 2013). The symptoms "may not necessarily be overtly manifested until several months or even a year after severe TBI" (Ponsford, 2013).

Whether or not TBI survivors could experience PTSD has been widely debated. Strictly speaking, PTSD requires that the one exposed to a traumatic event display reexperiencing symptoms, such as intrusive memories of the event or feeling that the event was recurring. TBI survivors often experience post-traumatic amnesia and, therefore, do not recall the specific event. The memory may have never been stored in the brain due to the impact of the injury. Some researchers explained the existence of PTSD by outlining specific criteria, such as experiencing distressing events associated with trauma that occurred either before or after the period of amnesia, processing the trauma by the limbic system at an implicit level of awareness, or learning of the trauma as told by others reconstructed the memory (Sciutella, 2007). Earlier views that PTSD could not develop in the presence of amnesia have given way to a recognition that mild TBI may instead increase the likelihood of the development of PTSD (Al-Ozairi et al., 2015). Al-Ozairi et al. (2015) state that reexperiencing and avoidant symptoms are most common among mild TBI survivors. However, Bryant (2001) has demonstrated that PTSD does occur with significant frequency following mild, moderate, and severe TBI. Several factors contribute to this new understanding, including implicit (unconscious) encoding of affective and sensory experiences (e.g., sights and smells) associated with the traumatic event, conscious encoding of some aspects of the event, reconstruction of the trauma memory from secondary sources (e.g., family, other observers), and memory of circumstances surrounding the event that may also be psychologically traumatic (e.g., sights at the scene after consciousness was regained; Vasterling et al., 2019). A related issue was the lack of emotional expression exhibited by TBI survivors. PTSD requires one to experience intense fear, helplessness, or horror related to the event. Stimulus revaluation speaks to this dilemma. Although the memory did not elicit strong human emotion, new information altered the

PTSD v.mTBI

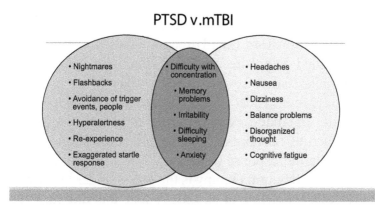

Figure 9.1 Comparative Symptoms of TBI and PTSD

representation of the trauma, dramatically increasing fear and perception of the threat (Harvey et al., 2005). Another explanation for the coexistence of PTSD and TBI is the dual-representation theory, which states that "some degree of consciousness is essential for the creation of any kind of trauma memory" (Harvey et al., 2005). Periods of impaired consciousness retained situationally accessible memory and formed the basis of reexperiencing sensations involved in the trauma. Coetzer (2018) explains the differences in similar symptomology of PTSD and TBI. He states that poor emotional expression in PTSD presents as emotional blunting versus the apathy of TBI. Memory loss with PTSD relates to the trauma itself instead of everyday memory loss of TBI (Coetzer, 2018). The overlapping of symptoms is depicted in Figure 9.1.

A thorough assessment identifying the similar and differentiating symptoms presents a clearer picture of what the client is experiencing and from what diagnosis.

Coping Strategies

The goal of treating PTSD is to eventually eliminate the symptoms. Ponsford (2013) recommends treating PTSD with graded exposure therapies that slowly confront the triggers that were previously sought to be avoided. Another recommendation is to encourage clients to speak about the traumatic event in order to reduce the symptoms, such as flashbacks, intrusive memories, and exaggerated startle response (Ponsford, 2013). In this writing, cognitive behavioral therapy is the gold standard for treating PTSD. Vasterling et al. (2019) state that although the research is in its "early stages, the available evidence suggests that cognitive behavioral therapy interventions commonly used to treat PTSD are both effective and safe in treating individuals with PTSD and TBI across a range of severities."

Narrative psychology was another preferred form of counseling with brain injury clients due to the focus of creating a life story. A major tenet of this approach is asking the client to makes sense of an experience as it pertains to the story of the world and his or her role in it. Smit (2006), a graduate of the University of Pretoria, highlights self-narratives as a means for TBI survivors to make sense of what happened to them. The construction of a new self-narrative helped create the sense of self, where they fit in the world and their purpose. Smit (2006) states that some of the "challenging behavior following brain injury could result from frustrated efforts to either reconstruct pre-injury self-narrative, or construct new preferred self-narratives." Most brain injury survivors in my practice, as they recover, long to create purpose from their pain. Writing a narrative of their post-injury self is a vehicle whereby they help other survivors and family members understand their recovery experience.

Faith and Hope

As a Christian counselor specializing in brain injury, I have found that many, if not all, of my clients who have suffered a brain injury lean on their faith as a coping strategy. Interestingly, they bring the topic of faith to the counseling experience, not me. From all kinds of backgrounds and all kinds of beliefs, their faith seems to alleviate some of the psychological effects of brain injury. In addressing depression, one client referred to King David in Psalm 42, where he says that he is worn out from groaning. He says that all night long, his bed is flooded with his tears. In addressing anxiety, many have reminded themselves to pray and meditate on the promises in the Bible, the Torah, or other spiritual books. One TBI survivor who suffered her injury in World War II at the hands of Josef Mengele in Auschwitz stated, "God has a purpose for me that I should live." Faith is an integral part of healing and recovery. Faith leads the survivor to search for their purpose. Another survivor said that after the injury, she longed to find her place in the world again. Her faith helped her get on that path of finding her place. She now speaks of her experience offering hope to others. Potentially, there is an opportunity for enhanced relationships, increased personal strength, new possibilities, life appreciation, and heightened spirituality (Klonoff, 2010).

During an informal conversation, Dr. Andrew Maas, a former neurosurgeon from Antwerp, Belgium, was asked what he thought about hope after brain injury. He quickly stated that "hope is as essential as breath." I have found that to be true in my practice. Both brain injury survivors and their family members long to know that there is hope for recovery, hope of creating a new life, hope that the suffering was not in vain. The emphasis on abilities and strengths versus disabilities and limitations is critical in the recovery process. Hope is embedded in this process. Collins and Kuehn (2004) state that "hope provides the individual with a positive option that negates the perceived rejection and failure, minimizes loss, and is differentiated from learned helplessness." Hope focuses on the belief that one's goals can be achieved in spite of obstacles (Collins & Kuehn, 2004). Acknowledging the limitations and deficits is also an opportunity to identify coping strategies that can assist in adaptation and recovery. Kortte et al. (2012) found that hopefulness during the rehabilitation process is related to positive psychological adjustment. The formation of purpose, personal growth, regaining identity, developing community, and hopefulness is the opportunity in brain injury recovery (Klonoff, 2010). Hope believes in the ability for every survivor to embrace that their life-changing event can create meaning and higher purpose. One of our beloved physical medicine and rehabilitation physicians recommended to her patients to adjust one's focus from inside to outside. In other words, turn one's attention to someone in need. This one action gives hope to one in need and purpose for the survivor. Whether one is a counselor, friend, family member, educator, physician, or therapist, communicating hope for recovery and purpose for the future gives the much-needed breath to keep going, to not give up, and to have faith.

References

Abbasi, J. (n.d.). Why friends make us happier, healthier people. *happify.com*. www.happify.com/hd/why-friends-make-us-happier/

Albrecht, J., Peters, M., Smith, G., & Rao, V. (2017). Anxiety and posttraumatic stress disorder among medicare beneficiaries after traumatic brain injury. *Journal of Head Trauma Rehabilitation, 32*, 178–184.

Al-Ozairi, A., McCullagh, S., & Feinstein, A. (2015). Predicting posttraumatic stress symptoms following mild, moderate, and severe traumatic brain injury: The role of posttraumatic amnesia. *Journal of Head Trauma Rehabilitation, 30*, 283–289.

American Psychiatric Association. (2013). *Diagnostic and statistical manual of mental disorders* (5th ed.). Author.

Arthur, M. (2021). *Looking for Eden* [Unpublished manuscript].

Ashman, T., Cantor, J., Tsaousides, T., Spielman, L., & Gordon, W. (2014). Comparison of cognitive behavioral therapy and supportive psychotherapy for the treatment of depression following traumatic brain injury: A randomized controlled trial. *Journal of Head Trauma Rehabilitation, 29*, 467–478.

Barker, K. (Ed.). (1985). *The NIV study Bible: New international version*. Zondervan.

Behn, N., Marshall, J., Togher, L., & Cruice, M. (2019). Setting and achieving individualized social communication goals for people with acquired brain injury (ABI) within a group treatment: Individualized social communication goals for people with ABI. *International Journal of Language & Communication Disorders, 54*, 828–840. https://doi.org/10.1111/1460-6984.12488

BibleGateway. (2015). *Holy Bible, new living translation*. www. biblegateway.com/versions/New-Living-Translation-NLT-Bible/ (Original work published 1996)

Bielinis, E., Jaroszewska, A., Łukowski, A., & Takayama, N. (2019). The effects of a forest therapy programme on mental hospital patients with affective and psychotic disorders. *International Journal of Environmental Research and Public Health, 17*(1), 118. https://doi.org/10.3390/ijerph17010118

Brand, J. E. (2015). The far-reaching impact of job loss and unemployment. *Annual Review of Sociology, 41*, 359–375. https://doi.org/10.1146/annurev-soc-071913-043237

Bryant, R. (2001). Posttraumatic stress disorder and traumatic brain injury: Can they co-exist? *Clinical Psychological Review, 21*, 931–948.

Coetzer, R. (2018). *Anxiety and mood disorders following traumatic brain injury: Clinical assessment and psychotherapy*. Routledge.

Collins, A., & Kuehn, M. (2004). The construct of hope in the rehabilitative process. *Rehabilitation Education, 18*, 175–183.

Collins, R., Pastorek, N., Sharp, A., & Kent, T. (2012). Behavioral and psychiatric comorbities of TBI. In J. Tsao (Ed.), *Traumatic brain injury: A clinician's guide to diagnosis, management, and rehabilitation* (pp. 223–244). Springer.

Crocq, M. A., & Crocq, L. (2000). From shell shock and war neurosis to posttraumatic stress disorder: A history of psychotraumatology. *Dialogues in Clinical Neuroscience, 2*(1), 47–55. https://doi.org/10.31887/DCNS.2000.2.1/macrocq

Douglas, J., & Spellacy, F. (2000). Correlates of depression in adults with severe traumatic brain injury and their carers. *Brain Injury, 14*, 71–88.

Duran, S. (2021, March 24). I miss my brain. *Facebook*. www.facebook.com/groups/108398302515255/posts/4046340278721018

Fides, B. N., Lane, J. C., Lenard, J., & Vulcan, A. P. (2020, February 23). Passenger cars and occupant injury: Side impact crashes. *Accident Research Centre*. www.monash.edu/muarc/archive/our-publications/reports/atsb134

Friedman, M. (n.d.). *PTSD history and overview*. US Department of Veterans Affairs. www.ptsd.va.gov/professional/treat/essentials/history_ptsd.asp

Gaines, C., Goff, S., Lambo, J., Matsumoto, M., Nguyen, L., Ross, R., Umetani, S. (Producers), & Ross, R. (Director). *The courage to run with chip Gaines and Gabe Grunewald* [Video file]. www.imdb.com/video/vi1106493465?playlistId=tt14411 796&ref_=tt_ov_vi

Gallo, L. (2015). *Speaking of psychology: The stress of money*. www.apa.org/research/action/speaking-of-psychology/financial-stress

Gardner, R. C., Dams-O'Connor, K., Morrissey, M. R., & Manley, G. T. (2018). Geriatric traumatic brain injury: Epidemiology, outcomes, knowledge gaps, and future directions. *Journal of Neurotrauma, 35*(7), 889–906. https://doi.org/10.1089/neu.2017.5371

Gomes-Osman, J., Cabral, D. F., Morris, T. P., McInerney, K., Cahalin, L. P., Rundek, T., Oliveira, A., & Pascual-Leone, A. (2018). Exercise for cognitive brain health in aging: A systematic review for an evaluation of dose. *Neurology: Clinical Practice, 8*(3), 257–265. https://doi.org/10.1212/CPJ.0000000000000460

Gronwall, D., Wrightson, P., & Waddell, P. (1998). *Head injury: The facts* (2nd ed.). Oxford University Press.

Harvey, A., Kopelman, M., & Brewin, C. (2005). PTSD and traumatic brain injury. In J. Vasterling & C. Brewin (Eds.) *Neuropsychology of PTSD: Biological, cognitive, and clinical perspectives* (pp. 230–248). Guilford Press.

Hawthorne, G., Gruen, R., & Kaye, A. (2009). Traumatic brain injury and long-term quality of life: Findings from an Australian study. *Journal of Neurotrauma, 26*, 1623–1633.

Hoofien, D., Gilboa, A., Vakil, E., & Donovick, P. (2001). Traumatic brain injury (TBI) 10–20 years later: A comprehensive outcome study of psychiatric symptomology, cognitive abilities and psychosocial functioning. *Brain Injury, 15*, 189–209.

Hoppen, T. H., & Morina, N. (2019). The prevalence of PTSD and major depression in the global population of adult war survivors: A meta-analytically informed estimate in absolute numbers. *European Journal of Psychotraumatology, 10*(1), 1578637. https://doi.org/10.1080/20008198.2019.1578637

Jones, M., & Jorge, R. (2019). Depression following TBI: Can it be prevented? *Psychiatric Times, 36,* 24–25.

Jorge, R. (2008). Mood and anxiety disorders following traumatic brain injury. *Psychiatric Times, 25,* 65.

Juengst, S., Kumar, R., Failla, M., Goyal, A., & Wagner, A. (2015). Acute inflammatory biomarker profiles predict depression risk following moderate to severe traumatic brain injury. *Journal of Head Trauma Rehabilitation, 30,* 207–218.

Klonoff, P. (2010). *Psychotherapy after brain injury: Principles and techniques.* Guilford Press.

Kortte, K., Stevenson, J., Hosey, M. Castillo, R., & Wegener, S. (2012). Hope predicts positive functional role outcomes in acute rehabilitation populations. *Rehabilitation Psychology, 57,* 248–255.

Kreutzer, J., Godwin, E., & Marwitz, J. (2010). *The truth about divorce after brain injury.* Traumatic Brain Injury—Virginia Commonwealth University. https://tbi.vcu.edu/media/tbi/nrc-articles/TruthAboutDivorceWinter2010.pdf

Marsh, N., Kersel, D., Havill, J., & Sleigh, J. (2002). Caregiver burden during the year following severe traumatic brain injury. *Journal of Clinical and Experimental Neuropsychology, 24,* 434–447.

McIntyre, A., Rice, D., Janzen, S., Mehta, S., Harnett, A., Caughlin, S., Sequeira, K., & Teasell, R. (2020). Anxiety, depression, and quality of life among subgroups of individuals with acquired brain injury: The role of anxiety sensitivity and experiential avoidance. *NeuroRehabilitation, 47,* 45–53.

McKee-Ryan, F., & Maitoza, R. (2014, September). *Job loss, unemployment, and families.* Oxford Handbooks Online. www.oxfordhandbooks.com/view/10.1093/oxfordhb/9780199764921.001.0001/oxfordhb-9780199764921-e-027

MEDIAmaker. (n.d.-a). *Headway—the brain injury association.* www.headway.org.uk/

MEDIAmaker. (n.d.-b). Returning to work. Headway—the brain injury association. *Headway.* www.headway.org.uk/about-brain-injury/individuals/practical-issues/returning-to-work/

Mental Health Foundation. (2018, June 26). *Post-traumatic stress disorder (PTSD)*. www.mentalhealth.org.uk/a-to-z/p/post-traumatic-stress-disorder-ptsd

Mind. (n.d.). How to manage stress. Mind, the mental health charity—help for mental health problems. *Mind*. www.mind.org.uk/information-support/types-of-mental-health-problems/post-traumatic-stress-disorder-ptsd-and-complex-ptsd/symptoms/

Muir, J. (2015). *John Muir—The mountains of California: The mountains are calling and I must go*. Wanderlust.

Nathan, A. A., & Mirviss, S. (1998). *Therapy techniques: Using the creative arts*. Idyll Arbor.

Oz, F. (Director). (1991). *What about Bob* [film]. Laura Ziskin.

Pálsdóttir, A.-M., Stigsdotter, U., Persson, D., Thorpert, P., & Grahn, P. (2017). The qualities of natural environments that support the rehabilitation process of individuals with stress-related mental disorder in nature-based rehabilitation. *Urban Forestry & Urban Greening, 29*. https://doi.org/10.1016/j.ufug.2017.11.016.

Perryman, K., Blisard, P., & Moss, R. (2019, January 1). Using creative arts in trauma therapy: The neuroscience of healing | Journal of mental health counseling. *Journal of Mental Health Counseling, 41*, 80–94. https://meridian.allenpress.com/jmhc/article-abstract/4/1/80//12241/Using-Creative-Arts-in-Trauma-Therapy-The?redirectedFrom=fulltext

Ponsford, J. (2013). Dealing with the impact of TBI on psychological adjustment and relationships. In J. Ponsford, S. Sloan, & P. Snow (Eds.) *Traumatic brain injury: Rehabilitation for everyday adaptive living* (2nd ed.). Psychology Press.

Poulsen, D. V., Stigsdotter, U. K., Djernis, D., & Sidenius, U. (2016). 'Everything just seems much more right in nature': How veterans with post-traumatic stress disorder experience nature-based activities in a forest therapy garden. *Health Psychology Open*. Advance online publication. https://doi.org/10.1177/2055102916637090

Qiu, M., Sha, J., & Utomo, S. (2020). Listening to forests: Comparing the perceived restorative characteristics of natural soundscapes before and after the COVID-19 pandemic. *Sustainability, 13*(1), 293. https://doi.org/10.3390/su13010293

Rousseau, I. (n.d.). Eden, trans J. M. Coetzee. *Poetry Magazine.* www.poetryfoundation.org/poetrymagazine/poems/49319/eden-56d22b4995df2

Ruff, R., & Jamora, C. (2008). Forensic neuropsychology and mild traumatic brain injury. *Psychological Injury and Law, 1,* 122–137.

Rush, B., Malec, J., Brown, A., & Moessner, A. (2006). Personality and functional outcome following traumatic brain injury. *Rehabilitation Psychology, 51,* 257–264.

Sciutella, A. (2007). Neuropsychiatry and traumatic brain injury. In J. Elbaum & D. Benson (Eds.) *Acquired brain injury: An intergrative neuro-rehabilitation approach.* Springer.

Siegel, D. J. (2020). *The developing mind: How relationships and the brain interact to shape who we are* (3rd ed.). Guilford Publications.

Smit, M. (2006). *A qualitative exploration of experiences of others and accounts of self in the narratives of persons who have experienced traumatic brain injury* (Unpublished master's thesis). University of Pretoria.

Stein, E. (2020). *Budding time too brief.* www.poemsinthewaitingroom.org/poems.html

Stuckey, H. L., & Nobel, J. (2010). The connection between art, healing, and public health: A review of current literature. *American Journal of Public Health, 100*(2), 254–263. https://doi.org/10.2105/AJPH.2008.156497

Tartakovsky, M. (2016, September 18). 7 ways to honor yourself every day. *Psych Central.* https://psychcentral.com/blog/7-ways-to-honor-yourself-every-day#1

The Myers & Briggs Foundation. (n.d.). *The Myers & Briggs Foundation—MBTI® basics.* www.myersbriggs.org/my-mbti-personality-type/mbti/basics

Tomberg, T., Toomela, A., Pulver, A., & Tikk, A. (2005). Coping strategies, social support, life orientation and health-related quality of life following traumatic brain injury. *Brain Injury, 19,* 1181–1190.

U.S. Department of Health and Human Services, National Institutes of Health, National Institute of Mental Health. (2015). *NIMH strategic plan for research* (NIH Publication No. 02–2650). www.nimh.nih.gov/about/strategic-planning-reports/index. shtml

Vasterling, J., Jacob, S., & Rasmusson, A. (2019). Posttraumatic stress disorder. In J. Silver, T. McAllister, & D. Arciniegas (Eds.) *Textbook of traumatic brain injury* (3rd ed.). American Psychiatric Association Publishing.

Index

Abbasi, Jennifer 22
accommodations 33, 36, 44, 51–52, 101
air circulation 71
aircraft technical malfunctions 100
Al-Ozairi, A. 144
American Psychological Association (APA) 95
anxiety 17, 22–23, 36, 38, 39, 49, 52, 71, 76, 79, 81, 94, 110–111, 113–114, 123, 131, 134, 139–143, 140

Best Personal Finance App 90
Bielinis, E. 113
blurry vision 49
body, healing of 43
body/soul/spirit, healing of 43
brain injury 22; categories of 55; cognitive abilities 50; communication with colleagues 64–65; communication with employer 63–64; conduct on-scene interviews 47; effects of 47; faith and hope 147–148; influential factors 63; physical condition of 57–58; psychological/social health 58–62; realistic attitude 63; returning to work 62–63; structured home program, suggestions for 65–66; support for making successful return to work 62; survivors of 62, 138, 146–147; symptoms 131; as ultimate disrupter 84; see also traumatic brain injury (TBI)
Brain Injury Association 61, 124
Brain Trauma Foundation 125
Brand, J. E. 89
broadcasting 29, 30, 33, 48
Bryant, R. 144

Camp Wolf, Kuwait 100–101
car accident 4, 25, 34, 87, 109, 111–112

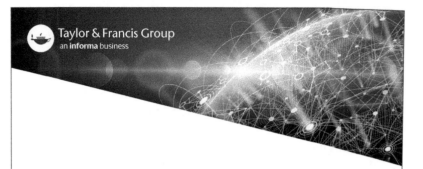

Taylor & Francis eBooks

www.taylorfrancis.com

A single destination for eBooks from Taylor & Francis with increased functionality and an improved user experience to meet the needs of our customers.

90,000+ eBooks of award-winning academic content in Humanities, Social Science, Science, Technology, Engineering, and Medical written by a global network of editors and authors.

TAYLOR & FRANCIS EBOOKS OFFERS:

A streamlined experience for our library customers

A single point of discovery for all of our eBook content

Improved search and discovery of content at both book and chapter level

REQUEST A FREE TRIAL
support@taylorfrancis.com

 Routledge
Taylor & Francis Group

 CRC Press
Taylor & Francis Group